T0137589

Once Upon a

Pose

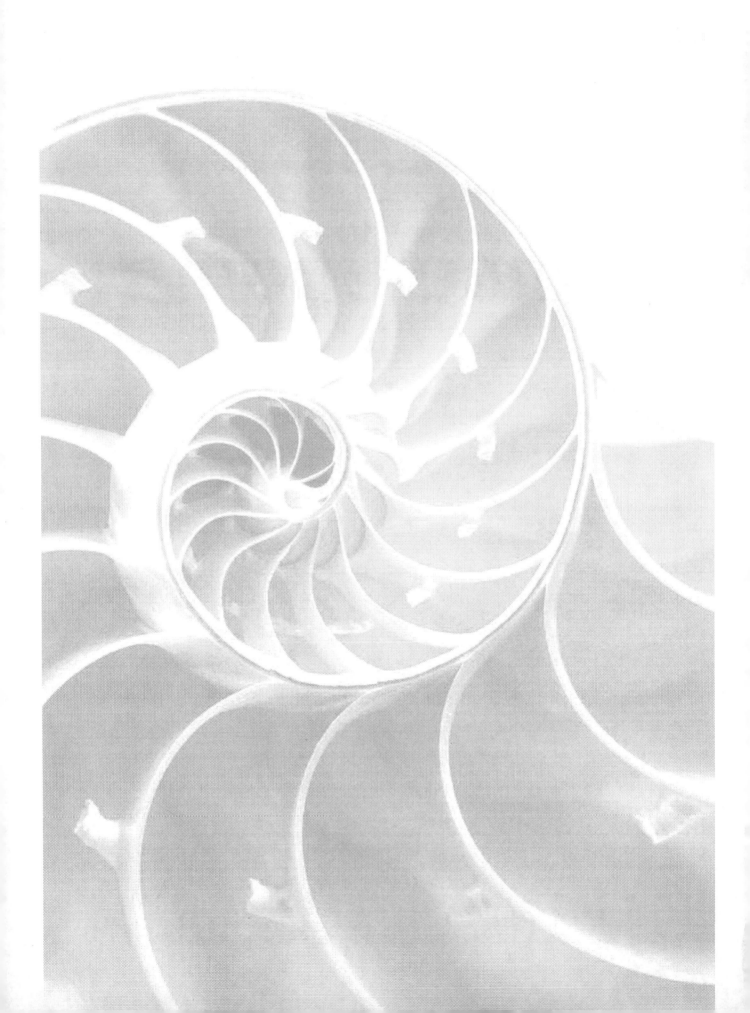

Once Upon a Pose

A Guide to Yoga Adventure Stories for Children

by Donna Freeman

The exercises in this book are gentle and safe, provided the instructions are followed carefully. This is not an exercise program, and is not intended to give specific health or medical advice. The publishers and author disclaim all liability in connection with the use of the information in individual cases. If you have any doubts as to the suitability of the exercises, consult a physician.

Order this book online at www.trafford.com
or email orders@trafford.com

Most Trafford titles are also available at major online book retailers.

Printed in Victoria, BC, Canada.

ISBN: 978-1-4269-2220-6

Library of Congress Control Number: 2009941109

Our mission is to efficiently provide the world's finest, most comprehensive book publishing service, enabling every author to experience success. To find out how to publish your book, your way, and have it available worldwide, visit us online at www.trafford.com

Trafford rev. 12/01/09

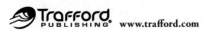 www.trafford.com

North America & international
toll-free: 1 888 232 4444 (USA & Canada)
phone: 250 383 6864 ♦ fax: 812 355 4082

For my children: may you be blessed with love, health,
friends, wealth, and most of all, time to enjoy them.

Acknowledgements

This project, like most others, wouldn't have been possible without the generous help and support of numerous individuals. I especially want to thank the staff at Leo Nickerson Elementary School in St Albert, Alberta for their support, assistance, and feedback. Also, I wish to extend a huge thank you to Lara Salm and Christian Laplante for their assistance with the French translations. Merci mille fois! I wish to acknowledge my friends and acquaintances who willingly offered their skills and knowledge, and made sure I didn't make too many mistakes: Kathy Nelson, Jodi Parrotta, Julie Visscher Rosenberger, Darlene Van Halst, and Lori Zastre. Many thanks to my hardworking and cheerful models, Alea, Ariana, Chloe, Drew, Elizabeth, Greer, Joshua, Madison, and Spencer. And mostly I want to thank my family who knew I could do this even when I didn't think it possible, and who endured neglect and a general state of chaos while I was engaged in research and writing. Sure do love you guys.

Foreword

I was thrilled that Freeman introduced such a comprehensive manual for yogis, students, and teachers everywhere.

I've been teaching yoga for over 15 years and wish this book was available when I started out. I've seen, over the years, what a tremendous difference yoga makes for children by enhancing body awareness, developing confidence, and teaching children breathing techniques to self calm. I've taught yoga to children who experienced severe abuse to mild ADD, and yet every child responds to yoga. Yoga develops a healthy mind because it taps all the senses, fuels the body with energy and releases tension so that children feel good. By moving the body in asanas, children release anxiety, anger, sadness and negative thoughts. When children think positively, their confidence and self esteem soars. Self esteem is so critical for a child, and it's our responsibility as a community to empower them. It also naturally causes loads of laughter which is so beneficial and healing.

Yoga philosophy maintains that a healthy spine creates balance and acts as a conduit to a sound mind. In a world where everyone is competing to be the best, yoga is about the individual thriving in a non-competitive environment. Children need a place to feel safe, where they will not be judged, and the yoga classroom provides this environment. With all the instant gratification today, children have little idea of waiting for something. Yoga teaches values like humility and patience that can be extremely beneficial to this generation. It has a humbling effect because there's always something you can't do.

The skills yoga embodies are life skills that can benefit them physically, emotionally and mentally throughout their life. I think every child should be taught yoga just to experience the sheer joyfulness of the spirit! Read this book in its entirety and gain great insight on how to playfully introduce yoga into the life of a child. It will change their life.

Namaste,

Mary Kaye Chryssicas

Preface

Many talented people have published works directed at yoga for children. For years I've used them, adapting and integrating the principles into my own version of teaching kids yoga.

I found that kids responded most favourably when I integrated yoga poses and philosophy into a story. Over the years I developed numerous story themes when working with elementary-aged children in classrooms, at summer camps, and for birthday parties. These stories helped give yoga a context that was easily followed, and provided a concrete meaning for the yoga postures. Children four to 12 years-old could understand the various settings and were able to use their imagination in a creative manner, developing their own personal story within the plot framework.

While giving a workshop at a teachers' convention, someone finally asked me to put my stories into a book so that the teachers could benefit more fully from the many ideas I was presenting. And so, the idea of a working resource specifically for use in classrooms was born.

Teachers want to use yoga in their schools to harness its many benefits and meet the daily physical activity requirements. However, application to the classroom is challenging and often requires additional preparation or yoga expertise in order to be successfully implemented. Being a teacher myself, I know how pressed for time these professionals are, and I wanted to provide a working resource to make bringing yoga into the classroom as easy as possible.

The principle purpose of this book is to help to bring the benefits of yoga to kids. It will provide a concise foundation of yoga theory focusing particularly on *Hatha* yoga. The relevance of yoga in the school setting will then be discussed, emphasizing physical activity and classroom application. Ten different stories will be presented with clear, step-by-step directions on how to perform the various yoga postures. Breathing and relaxation will also be covered, and their importance examined. Finally, various games and activities will be introduced for those who want to 'play' yoga.

I am a firm believer in the need to bring the many benefits of yoga to our children. Its unique capacity to adapt to the individual's physical abilities and emotional needs— while fully supporting personal growth and individuality in a non-competitive manner— is desperately needed by teachers and students alike. Here is a fun and fully interactive way to explore our world, expand our abilities, learn lifelong habits of health and vitality, and create something new and beautiful with each practice.

I hope you will take this opportunity to bring yoga adventure stories into your classroom. As you do, enjoy the journey and the laughter.

Namaste,

Donna Freeman

Contents

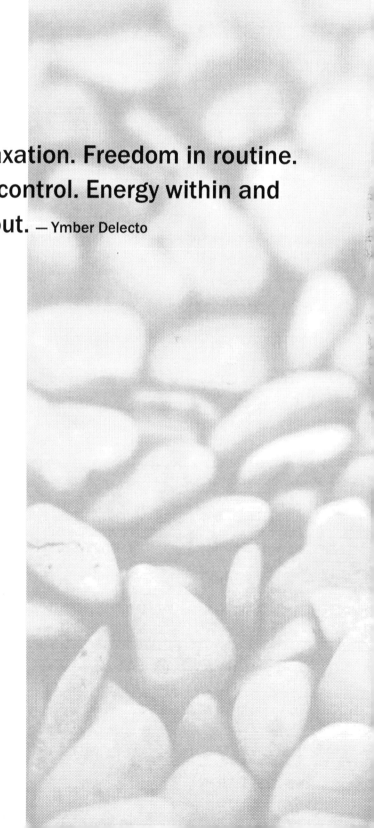

Chapter 1   Yoga 101

Yoga is invigoration in relaxation. Freedom in routine. Confidence through self-control. Energy within and energy without. — Ymber Delecto

Yoga Foundations

The word *Yoga* comes from the Sanskrit word *yuj* meaning 'yoke' or 'union.' When you join the **body** with the **breath** and the **mind**, then you are doing yoga. Yoga can be practised by anyone—regardless of physical ability—as long as there is a union among these three elements. This book focuses on *Hatha* yoga. The meaning of *hatha* is derived from the syllables *ha* meaning "sun" and *tha* meaning "moon." *Hatha* yoga is the union of the sun and the moon, a healthy joining of two opposites—the mind and body—which leads to strength, vitality, and tranquility.

Hatha yoga is essentially physical yoga, and involves various postures or poses (*asanas*), breathing exercises (*pranayama*), and relaxation. There are numerous other types of yoga including *Jnana* yoga (study and meditation), *Bhakti* yoga (prayer), *Karma* yoga (selfless actions), *Mantra* yoga (sacred sounds), and *Raja* yoga (Eight Limbs—*Yoga Sutras*).

The greatest classical text from the yoga school of Indian philosophy is the *Yoga Sutras* by Patañjali, written in the second century BC. These 'threads' on yoga are condensed nuggets of wisdom, stating concisely—and often precisely—essential points or techniques. Originally these teachings were oral and were easily memorized, recited or chanted. Their teachings, however, are profound enough to provide hours of discussion, and a lifetime of contemplation.

The Eight Limbs of *Raja* yoga (as explained in the *Yoga Sutras*) may have been written thousands of years ago, but they apply as much today as they did then. They need not be practised in a particular order, as they are interdependent. As you learn the postures, your breath control and concentration improve. These skills will hopefully assist in living basic observances and restraints of conduct. The limbs essentially intertwine to lead us to our ultimate goal of self-realization, or *Samadhi*.

There are numerous styles of yoga currently practised. However, all of the styles share a common lineage. The founders of three major styles—Ashtanga, Iyengar and Viniyoga—were all students of Sri Krishnamacharya, a famous teacher at the

---

EIGHT LIMBS OF YOGA

Yama:	restraints
Niyama:	observances
Asana:	postures
Pranayama:	breath control
Pratyahara:	sense withdrawal
Dharana:	concentration
Dhyana:	meditation
Samadhi:	self-realization

Yoga Institute at the Mysore Palace in India. Two other styles, Integral and Sivananda, were created by disciples of the famous guru Sivananda. The following is a list of styles and a brief explanation of each. No style is better than another; it's simply a matter of personal preference.

Ananda – Ananda yoga is a classic style using *asana* and *pranayama* to awaken the body. It is a gentle practice, focusing on the subtle energies within oneself and on affirmations.

Anusara – Anusara was developed by John Friend, and is a heart-opening, spiritually inspiring practice, which also deeply respects alignment and students' abilities and limitations.

Ashtanga – Developed by K. Pattabhi Jois, Ashtanga is a physically demanding, serious workout involving flows, jumps and breathing techniques to develop strength, flexibility and stamina. Power Yoga is derived from Ashtanga.

Bikram – Bikram Choudhury developed this hot style of yoga, which follows 26 *asanas* that help warm and stretch muscles, tendons and ligaments. Many Hot Yoga classes are inspired by this style.

Integral – Integral yoga puts almost as much emphasis on breathing and meditation as on postures. It was developed by Swami Satchidananda, and is used in *Dr. Dean Ornish's Program to Reversing Heart Disease*.

Iyengar – B.K.S. Iyengar's popular style is noted for its attention to specific alignment and detail. The use of props (belts, blocks, blankets, etc.) is often used to achieve proper alignment.

Kripalu – With an emphasis on breath, alignment, and coordinating the breath with movement, students of Kripalu yoga focus on their physical and psychological reactions to yoga postures.

Kundalini – Focusing on a controlled release of Kundalini energy, this style involves poses, breath, coordination of breath and movement, as well as meditation.

Sivananda – Developed by Vishnu-devananda, Sivananda yoga follows a set structure that includes *pranayama*, classic *asanas*, and relaxation. Vishnu-devananda wrote one of the contemporary yoga classics, *The Complete Illustrated Book of Yoga*.

Svaroopa – Opening the spine from the tail bone to the top, Rama Berch has developed a significantly different way of doing yoga. This is not an athletic practice, but strives for an inner experience with greater consciousness.

Viniyoga – This is the approach developed by Sri T. Krishnamacharya, where function is stressed over form. Personal practices are taught privately with a focus on *asana*, flow of breath, movement of the spine, sequencing and adaptations, as necessary.

Yoga Language

The original language of yoga is Sanskrit, a classical language of South Asia, and one of the official languages of India. It has influenced many modern-day Asian languages, and is akin to Latin or Greek in European languages. English translations of Sanskrit are somewhat cumbersome, and will be too heavy for most children.

However, teaching the names of poses can be an interesting cultural and linguistic endeavour, and may open students' eyes to the world beyond their community. For that purpose, Sanskrit names are provided for each pose. The two words most commonly used in relation to yoga are *namaste* and *aum*.

Namaste is a form of greeting or salutation, which, translated literally, means 'I bow to you.' When spoken to another person, it is commonly accompanied by a slight bow made with hands pressed together, palms touching and fingers pointed upwards, in front of the chest (**Prayer** position): the higher the hands, the more reverence and respect shown. The gesture can also be performed wordlessly and carry the same meaning. Yoga students generally repeat *namaste* at the end of a yoga session to express appreciation for sharing and growing together.

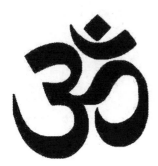

Aum is a combination of the first and last letters of the Sanskrit alphabet. It is said to symbolically encompass all the sounds of the universe. In effect, it is the beginning and the end, the alpha and omega of the yogic language. It is often used as a basis for chanting and meditation; properly performing *Aum* helps center and calm yoga participants, bringing a sense of peace and connection to the universe.

Yoga Philosophy

Teachers may encounter a knee-jerk reaction to introducing yoga in their school or classroom from parents who mistakenly fear religious or moral instruction contrary to their own beliefs. Many teachers are shocked to learn of this negative reaction, seeing the many benefits yoga can bring to the classroom. Still, it is my experience, and the news headlines agree, that some groups or individuals may feel uncomfortable with teaching yoga to young, impressionable children. There are aspects of yoga which do delve into the spiritual realm, making yoga a truly holistic life practice. However, the school environment is not the place for this instruction, and you can assure your parents that the focus will be on *Hatha* or physical yoga.

Aum

Sit cross-legged, place your hands on your knees in *gyan mudra* (thumb and index finger forming a circle, other fingers elongated). *Aum* is generally considered to have 3½ measures: A, U, M and silence. Close your eyes, inhale, then exhale as you perform *Aum*, repeating three times. The sound ahhhh starts in our chest at the heart center, moves upward with the ooooo sound in the throat center, and ends with the sound mmmmm, which vibrates the higher centers in the head.

For your convenience, I have included a one-page letter which you may photocopy and send to parents informing them that yoga will be taught in your classroom (see page 115 **Letter to Parents**). Hopefully, this will answer their questions and ease any concerns they may have regarding the stories in this book and how yoga will be presented to their children.

If there is a desire or interest to pursue the spiritual side of the practice, numerous resources and avenues are available for personal enrichment, with most being readily available in local libraries, bookstores, and yoga studios. The yoga association of your geographical area is often one of the best resources for finding certified teachers and yoga studios willing to assist in developing a personal yoga practice.

That being said, a basic understanding of the *yamas* and *niyamas*—the *dos* and *don'ts* of yoga—is necessary, and will help calm fears of the unknown. These tenets correspond to basic values of society. Teaching children these ethics helps them learn respect for themselves and others, as well as an appreciation for the world in which they live.

Yamas – Restraints
Living well in the world

Ahimsa – non-violence: an attitude of not wanting to harm anyone or anything, including yourself, in work, thought or action; another way to phrase it is to live with peace, kindness, and love.

Satya – honesty: being true to and honest with yourself and those you encounter; this includes speech and action, and leads to the development of trust and integrity.

Asteya – not stealing: take and use only that which is freely given, including physical possessions, ideas, and time; do not indulge in jealousy or coveting, knowing that you have enough.

Brahmacarya – conservation: controlling your senses, avoiding over-indulgences, refusing to let your desires diminish or disrespect anyone, including yourself; this means exercising self-control in all areas of life, including sexual, physical, and emotional.

Aparigraha – avoiding greed: do not hoard possessions, learn to distinguish want from need, and live off what you need, be it objects, food, time, or attention; learning to live simply and in agreement with the environment.

Niyamas – Observances
Learning about yourself

Saucha – cleanliness: taking care to have a clean body and environment, including good hygiene, a clean room and home, eating fresh, healthy food, and developing a life based on a foundation of pure actions, words and thoughts.

Santosha – contentment: being happy with who you are, where you are, and with what you have; living simply and frugally, cultivating a calm attitude, and learning to accept that what you have is enough.

Tapas – self-discipline: making the most of yourself, setting goals and not giving up easily; making a concerted effort, developing habits of hard work and perseverance; committing to something and sticking with it.

Svadhyaya – worthwhile study and learning: self-study and personal contemplation; lifelong learning and being open to new ideas and approaches; doing homework and investigating subjects of personal interest.

Ishvara pranidhana – surrender: letting go of preconceived notions of self, others, and situations; contemplating and committing to a higher power or divinity; living with love and recognizing the positive energy in life.

Yoga Props

Anything used to do yoga—other than your body, breath, and mind—is a prop. They are used primarily to assist individuals in learning and performing poses.

Props include but are not limited to:

MATS: yoga mats are very common, and are often considered the basic equipment necessary for yoga practice

BLOCKS: foam or wood blocks in varying sizes assist with alignment

STRAPS: long narrow straps assist with flexibility and alignment

BOLSTERS: various sizes and shapes of firm pillows help with deep relaxation and sometimes meditation

BLANKETS: blankets are used for alignment, comfort, and relaxation

CHAIRS: chairs support and expand pose variations

Props, however, are not essential to a safe and fulfilling yoga practice. In the school setting, mats are wonderful, and definitely help students define their personal space, making class management easier. Yoga mats are ideal, of course, but budget constraints may prohibit some schools from adding these to their available resources.

With that in mind, standard Physical Education mats already in use in the school are perfectly acceptable, as long as they are not too slippery. Another option is to work on a clean carpet. Gymnasiums, libraries, drama rooms, music rooms, and classrooms all make ideal locations to practise yoga. Teaching students to respect their body, its limitations and abilities, and to work at a safe level while performing any pose, is more important than the props used to assist in that endeavour.

Yoga is performed with bare feet. Shoes, while necessary for many cardio exercises, impede intimate understanding of the foot. Often we stick our feet into shoes and then forget about them entirely. Stretching and lengthening the toes, arches, heels and ankles are integral to a well-grounded yoga practice. As these areas are strengthened and stretched, the foot is healthier—better prepared to play its vital function in our lives. Balance is also keenly affected by footwear and bare feet allow a true understanding of the body's relationship to the earth.

Socks are also removed for safety as they can be slippery. Some students, however, have foot conditions and so, for health and sanitary reasons, socks should be allowed. Please stress, when this is the case, that safety comes first, and keep in mind that poses may need to be modified to prevent slips and injuries.

Props are fun to use and can definitely aid individuals in learning poses and proper alignment; lack of props, however, should not prevent anyone from trying yoga. Poses can always be modified to suit the environment in which they are practised. In effect, props should never be more important than the yoga.

Chapter 2   How to Use Yoga

You can teach a student a lesson for a day; but if you can teach him to learn by creating curiosity, he will continue the learning process as long as he lives. — Clay P. Bedford

Physical Activity

Children need physical activity. It is essential for the healthy development of their bodies to move, stretch, and challenge themselves physically. Children are encouraged to run, jump, play sports, explore the local park or playground, and engage in many different physical activities to develop physically, mentally, and emotionally into well-rounded adults.

Unfortunately, many of today's children and youth do not get even the minimum amount of activity required to fully meet these basic developmental demands. Our lifestyle is increasingly sedentary. Children—especially urban, western children—are much less active than they used to be, spending time in front of the television or computer and being driven in a car or bus. Add to this the North American diet, and we have a growing population of children and youth who are overweight and at risk of disease.

In answer to this societal epidemic, greater emphasis on health and physical activity in the schools has become paramount. The provincial governments of Ontario, Alberta and British Columbia have all introduced a Daily Physical Activity (DPA) requirement into the curriculum for school-aged children. This initiative aims to increase students' health and fitness levels through a minimum of 20-30 minutes of physical activity daily. The guiding principle behind this initiative recognizes the necessity for lifelong habits of physical activity and healthy lifestyles. These habits are most effectively taught while children are young, receptive, and in the process of developing lifestyle attitudes.

> **Health is a state of complete harmony of the body, mind and spirit. When one is free from physical disabilities and mental distractions, the gates of the soul open.** — B.K.S. Iyengar

The onus now is on implementation, which makes classroom teachers responsible for developing the habits of healthful living crucial to the proper physical, mental, and emotional development of our children. To

this end, programs such as Ever Active Schools (visit everactive.org) and Action Schools BC (visit www.actionschoolsbc.ca) have been developed as supports to implement positive lifestyle habits in the classroom. Many teachers, however, struggle with this mandate, finding it one more thing to add to their already extensive 'to do' list.

Benefits of Yoga Practice

Offering a fun, non-competitive, and easy way to involve all children in physical activities, as well as fulfill the DPA initiative, yoga can provide children with a foundation of physical fitness, personal discovery, and respect for self, others, and the environment, which will serve them well throughout their lives.

I have found children to be especially receptive to trying yoga. It is usually something different and exciting, with a hint of mystery. They want to learn to *Aum* and love to try the poses, often surprised at their newfound skills. Of course, they always request again and again, "that lying down, sleeping pose" (**Corpse** pose) when they get to forget their worries and concerns and can relax, breathe, and simply *be*.

Yoga is an ancient practice developed through observation and improvement of the connection between body, breath, and mind. Recently, scientific research has begun to document the many positive aspects and health benefits of yoga *asana* and *pranayama*. These benefits can be seen after just one yoga session, and are augmented with regular practice. Yoga is different from other forms of exercise, stressing quality of movement over quantity. A consistent *Hatha* yoga practice can quiet the mind and refresh the body, bringing health, relaxation, and happiness.

Yoga promotes strength, flexibility, good coordination and posture, as well as teaching children how to relax, concentrate, and be quiet and still. Yoga is a gentle, non-competitive form of exercise, and can be practised by children of varying ages and physical abilities without anyone feeling inadequate or inferior. Yoga is not about attaining perfect poses or 'being the best'— it is about learning to do what is right for your own body. Success is not measured against others, but against oneself.

Yoga helps children learn about their body and how it works. *Asanas* are fun while providing a challenge, and can be adapted to suit bodies of all ages and physical abilities. As *asanas* are easily demonstrated and repeated, children can learn yoga by observation and imitation—their primary method of learning. Properly taught and practised yoga *asanas* provide children with sound physical and mental health, and lead to balanced growth and development.

The benefits of yoga are extensive. Included here is a brief overview of some of these benefits and how they apply to children and the classroom setting.

Yoga Increases Flexibility

Yoga teaches you how to safely stretch your muscles. This releases the lactic acid that builds up with muscle use and which, without stretching, can result in stiffness, tension, pain, and fatigue. When opposing muscle groups are trained together, flexibility increases rapidly as the muscles groups work in unison, not against or without each other. Yoga also increases the range of motion in joints. Yoga stretches not only your muscles, but all of the soft tissues of your body, including ligaments and tendons. Children are naturally flexible, and are shown how to maintain this physical state while exploring various other areas for improvement.

> **Yogic exercises and breathing exercises, right and simple living and high thinking and meditation are important requisites for the preservation of health, for the attainment of the high standard of vigour and vitality, longevity and everlasting peace and joy.**
> — Swami Sivananda

Yoga Develops Strength and Resiliency

Muscle tone throughout the body is improved by requiring you to support your body weight in new ways, including standing poses, balance poses, and inversions. Nearly all poses build core strength, an integral aspect of a healthy body. Yoga focuses on developing long, strong muscles. Many *asanas* also involve muscle control, actively recruiting large and small muscles, and holding poses making it a challenging full body workout. In addition, a regular yoga practice improves the immune system through detoxification. It renews, invigorates, and heals the body. Both energy levels and endurance increase.

Yoga Improves Balance

Yoga creates balance and symmetry throughout the body: right and left, front and back, high and low. Imbalance creates pain and dysfunction, and can cause injury. Numerous *asanas* focus expressly on balancing on one leg at a time (e.g., **Tree**, **Eagle**, **Dancer**). Young children are just developing this ability and love to practise, while older children become quite adept at this skill and appreciate learning how to increase the difficulty level. People who practise yoga also seek mental and emotional balance in their daily lives. Learning when to push, control, and be assertive and when to yield, submit, and be passive, is part of the yoga experience.

Yoga Requires Concentration

Yoga focuses on the *now,* which develops focus, concentration, and discipline. This translates into increased attention span, memory, and learning efficiency, leading to improved academic achievement. Due to its attentive nature yoga helps train the mind and builds attention to detail. This training is augmented by mindfully performing breathing exercises and meditation. Many *asanas* also improve hand-eye coordination, reaction time, dexterity, and fine motor skills. Guided relaxation induces the relaxation response allowing the body to release and let go of stress while the mind focuses, helping to define and fulfill personal destiny.

Yoga Improves Breathing

Most forms of yoga emphasize deepening and lengthening the breath. Yogic breathing techniques, even when used short-term, increase chest wall expansion and forced expiratory lung volumes. Because of the deep, mindful breathing that yoga involves, lung capacity often improves and respiratory efficiency increases. This in turn can improve sports performance and endurance as well as provide release for people with asthma. See **Chapter #5 Breathing** (p.101) for an in-depth discussion and exercises.

Yoga Raises Body-Awareness and Self-Image

Doing yoga will give you an increased awareness of your own body. Yoga requires specific placement of body parts as well as small, subtle movements to improve your alignment. Over time, this will increase your level of comfort with your own body and develop spatial awareness and understanding. This, along with a longer, stronger body thanks to improved muscle tone, can lead to better posture and greater self-confidence. Teaching *asanas* also involves teaching basic anatomy which helps children understand and appreciate their bodies. Yoga generates a sense of peace and contentment, while enriching personal awareness and teaching self-acceptance.

Yoga Reduces Stress

There are numerous anti-stress benefits from yoga. The 'flight-or-flight response' is a normal reaction to external stimulus and perceived threats. However, modern day living often does not allow for a physical release of this response which can cause negative physiological and psychological effects. Yoga counters these effects by first decreasing the hormones and neurotransmitters produced in response to stress. This creates a feeling of calm. Second, there is an increase in 'feel good' hormones such as oxytocin, which is associated with feeling relaxed and connected to others. As a result, mood improves and subjective well-being increases. Third, yoga promotes calm, clear thinking, even in situations that call for fast reactions. See **Chapter #6 Relaxation** (p.105) for an in-depth discussion and exercises.

Yoga is Practical

Yoga is easy, low cost, and accessible. This is ideal for the school setting where cost is often a consideration in program implementation. It is non-competitive, as you slow down and work with your own experience. Everyone can do yoga and feel good about it. *Asanas* are easily adapted to accommodate any physical ability or limitation. See **Yoga for Special Needs**. (p.19) Furthermore, it can be practised anywhere with little or no equipment. In addition a yoga session can vary in time according to the demands of the day. A five minute relaxation session or 30 minute workout are both effective and practical.

Classroom Applications

Educators know that retention and true understanding increase as more senses are involved in the learning process. Ever since the development of the Myers Briggs Type Indicator during WWII, there has been great interest and debate regarding psychological preferences and cognitive style. One underlying theme, however, is present: people demonstrate various strengths and weaknesses in the ways they acquire, retain, and organize information.

Individuals may prefer concrete experiences or abstract theories, use reflective observation more often than active experimentation, or tend toward random or sequential organization patterns. Knowing your favoured style allows you to capitalize on strengths and adapt the learning process and techniques to greater advantage. Furthermore, learning-styles theories continually support the integration of various approaches in order for learning to be most effective.

Eight Intelligences

Verbal/Linguistic
Logical/Mathematical
Visual/Spatial
Body/Kinaesthetic
Musical/Rhythmic
Interpersonal
Intrapersonal
Naturalist

Marsha Wenig's YogaKids program (visit www.yogakids.com) is based on the eight intelligences all people exhibit as explained in Howard Gardner's Multiple Intelligence Theory, developed in 1983. Ms. Wenig's work demonstrates how the eight intelligences relate to yoga, and how basic *asanas* can stimulate multiple intelligences simultaneously.

> **You don't understand anything until you learn it more than one way.**
> — Marvin Minsky

The stories developed for this book explore and expand the concept of multiple intelligences and the integration of learning styles. They apply directly to numerous curriculum requirements for Grades K-6. Teachers can enrich and enliven classes and reap all the benefits of doing yoga with their students, while knowing they are directly supporting educational goals and helping all students to achieve governmental standards of education.

Yoga can be applied in all subjects, and can promote greater learning by simultaneously incorporating numerous abilities and senses. Involving more senses in learning results in increased integration of experiences and retention of the acquired knowledge. One example of this is to discuss the unique qualities of camels using a photo of a camel, then perform camel pose in the story **Trip Down the Nile** (p.44). In doing so, you have engaged verbal, visual, body, and even naturalist intelligences. I've found that children will remember a pose even two years later, with no re-enforcement during that time, after having taught yoga using a story. The contextual nature of the stories and the kinaesthetic performance of the *asanas* work hand-in-hand to support learning and retention.

The following pages include an itemized listing of some of the ways yoga supports various topics of study. They are divided into subject area for ease of reference, but most overlap, fulfilling multiple requirements simultaneously. Yoga truly rises to the challenge of being a physical activity which reinforces and enlarges the classroom experience.

Preschool and Kindergarten

CITIZENSHIP AND IDENTITY

- Celebrate individuality and unique gifts and talents
- Examine what makes them unique as individuals
- Participate in and contribute to group activities and partner poses
- Explore the history and geography of the community and the world
- Value personal stories as a means to belonging
- Create a climate of cooperation with partner poses and group activities
- Demonstrate respect for self and others

CREATIVE EXPRESSION

- Explore self-expression through movement and music
- Become aware of various forms of expression

NUMERACY

- Identify and create patterns using the poses

LITERACY

- Follow one- and two-step instructions
- Story writing: create a story in small groups using a few suggested poses
- Reading: read the literature suggestions given for each story. If there is not a pose for a particular page, have children create one
- Recite rhymes and sing songs
- Develop listening skills

PHYSICAL AND WELL-BEING

- Learn about basic body maintenance: deep breathing; providing water and nutrition; sleep and rest to heal and grow; cleanliness; exercise
- Develop attitudes and behaviours to promote a healthy lifestyle and wellness
- Increase locomotor, non-locomotor, and fine motor skills

PERSONAL AND SOCIAL

- Demonstrate positive relationships with others
- Contribute to group activities
- Demonstrate and practise independence

Division I (Grades 1-3)

ENGLISH LANGUAGE ARTS

- Participate in and contribute to group activities and partner poses
- Discuss traditions found in stories and texts
- Story writing: create a story in small groups using a few suggested poses
- Be exposed to different ways of interpreting stories and ideas
- Relate own ideas to new understandings and situations
- Develop listening skills
- Explain personal preferences and favourites
- Celebrate individuality and unique gifts and talents
- Write in journals before, during or after poses

MATHEMATICS

- Patterns: make patterns using the poses
- Group poses according to type: standing pose, balance pose, forward bend, back bend, twist, inversion, relaxation
- Collect data regarding class ability or pose difficulty
- Measure personal space in various poses (standing, seated, relaxation)

SOCIAL STUDIES

- Explore cultural undertones; for example, **Warrior** pose—a Masai warrior is very different from an English knight or a Samarai
- Explore the history and geography of the community and the world
- Explore the Family: meanings and relationships

SCIENCE

- Life cycle: examine flow and cycles of nature
- Biology: learn the functions of the skeleton, major muscle groups, and organs
- Anatomy: increase understanding of body parts and function, need for physical exercise, proper breathing, water, rest, and relaxation

PHYSICAL EDUCATION

- Learn about basic body maintenance: deep breathing; providing water and nutrition; sleep and rest to heal and grow; cleanliness; exercise
- Celebrate individuality and unique gifts and talents
- Participate at a personal level in a physical ability
- Develop and apply age-appropriate skills
- Play and work cooperatively in a non-competitive environment
- Work within the safe zone, understanding under- and over-exertion

- Experience fitness skills such as strength, flexibility, endurance, and balance

HEALTH AND LIFE SKILLS

- Celebrate individuality and unique gifts and talents
- Participate in and contribute to group activities and partner poses
- Explore self-expression through movement, becoming aware of various forms of expression
- Develop respect for self and others
- Develop trust, coordination, cooperation, and team building through partner poses and group activities
- Engage in positive strategies for stress management
- Learn safe and appropriate ways to share and express feelings
- Increase body awareness, impacting self-esteem, personal hygiene, positive coping strategies, and social behaviours

FOREIGN LANGUAGE

- Study each story's French translation
- Be introduced to Sanskrit terms and vocabulary

ART

- Gain knowledge of creativity and beauty, that each pose forms beautiful natural lines, curves and forms
- Visual arts: draw or photograph yoga or what the poses bring to mind

MUSIC

- Explore music through story musical suggestions

DRAMA

- Perform a personal story using yoga poses

Division II (Grades 4-6)

ENGLISH LANGUAGE ARTS

- Create narratives from personal experiences using yoga poses
- Story writing: create a story in small groups using a few suggested poses
- Journalling: ask questions (How are you feeling now? What does this pose bring to mind?) before, during and after yoga poses which students then journal
- Comprehend texts from various cultural traditions
- Communicate effectively to express ideas and opinions
- Use talk, notes, and personal writing to explore own and others' ideas
- Work cooperatively in group settings

MATHEMATICS

- Area: measure and compare each student's personal size and space doing various poses
- Use positional terms to describe movement
- Geometry: study the natural lines, angles, curves and arches created by your skeleton; learn proper alignment to protect your body and keep the nervous system, skeleton, and muscles strong and flexible
- Right angles: watch for proper alignment; shoulder blades and hips form horizontal lines parallel to each other; arms at shoulder height are perpendicular to the earth; visualize the lines your skeleton makes

- Explore patterns and relations in poses

SOCIAL STUDIES

- Explore cultural undertones; for example, **Warrior** pose—a Masai warrior is very different from an English knight or a Samarai
- Explore the history and geography of the community and the world

SCIENCE

- Life cycle: examine flow and cycles of nature
- Study the body as a machine: bones or limbs are the levers that move at the joints or fulcrums to lift and move your body
- Physics: apply natural laws of gravity, balance of force and energy to develop the body
- Examine the use of energy in yoga: gravitational (earth), electromagnetic (brain), chemical (oxygen), elastic (stretching and compressing), mechanical (body moving as a machine)
- Apply Newton's Laws of Motion: forces occur in equal and opposite pairs, action/reaction
- Apply Newton's Law of Gravity: your body is the machine that applies the forces to move your body of mass against the force of gravity coming from the earth
- Explore the sun, moon, and stars

- Investigate and interpret **Tree** pose
- Biology: examine the function of the skeleton, major muscle groups, and organs
- Anatomy: increase understanding of body parts and function, need for physical exercise, proper breathing, water, rest, and relaxation

PHYSICAL EDUCATION

- Learn basic body maintenance: deep breathing; providing water and nutrition; sleep and rest to heal and grow; cleanliness; exercise
- Learn practices that promote an active healthy lifestyle
- Celebrate individuality and unique gifts and talents
- Participate at a personal level in a physical ability
- Develop and apply age-appropriate skills
- Play and work cooperatively in a non-competitive environment
- Work within the safe zone, understanding under- and over-exertion
- Experience fitness skills such as strength, flexibility, endurance, balance
- Develop trust, coordination, cooperation, and team building through partner poses and group activities
- Participate in and contribute to group activities and partner poses

HEALTH AND LIFE SKILLS

- Learn safe and appropriate ways to share and express feelings
- Increase body awareness, impacting self-esteem, personal hygiene, positive coping strategies, social behaviours, emotional wellness
- Explore self-expression through movement, becoming aware of various forms of expression
- Develop respect for self and others
- Engage in positive strategies for stress management
- Evaluate the need for balance and variety in daily activities

FOREIGN LANGUAGE

- Study each story's French translation
- Be introduced to Sanskrit terms and vocabulary

ART

- Gain knowledge of creativity and beauty, that each pose forms beautiful natural lines, curves and forms
- Visual arts: draw or photograph yoga or what the poses bring to mind

MUSIC

- Explore music through story musical suggestions
- Choreograph a yoga sequence (Yoga Dance)

DRAMA

- Perform a personal story using yoga poses

Yoga Clubs

An extra-curricular yoga club may be just what is needed in your school. I've seen yoga clubs that run once a week, twice a month, or monthly, all with great success. You may also want to consider a finite club that meets for a certain number of weeks or months (January through March, for instance) instead of throughout the entire year. There are lots of options and variations. It's simply a matter of finding something that works for you and your school.

Yoga clubs provide a wonderful opportunity to explore yoga in more detail than you may have opportunity to in the classroom. This may be the perfect venue to delve into and explore partner poses, yoga activities, yoga games, and self-reflection through meditation or journalling. A yoga club may also become a selling point for your school as an interesting and diverse option when students consider where to enrol.

A few things to consider before embarking on a yoga club are:

Do you have the time? A yoga club will require the typical extra-curricular devotion of most other clubs. What you put into it is what you get out. Ask yourself if your commitments (personal and professional) allow you the time to sponsor a club.

Is there sufficient interest for a club? Is there a core of interested individuals who will show up and put off other interests to come to yoga during their personal time? I've taught a yoga club where participants paid a small fee to get on the list but still didn't show up because of conflicting interests or a lack of commitment. If you're putting in the time and effort, make sure the students are dedicated as well. Otherwise, be prepared to offer the club as a service for whoever shows up. Be forewarned that yoga clubs often become hugely popular as word gets out about how great the kids feel afterwards.

Where will you meet? A music room, drama room, fitness room, gym, or classroom are perfect locations for a yoga club. Be sure that the space is available for your scheduled club dates. Having one location will make it easier to meet with students instead of bouncing around the school to find available space each time.

Do you know enough or are you bringing in a yoga instructor? The yoga expertise required for a club is higher than when doing it in a classroom setting. Are you comfortable with your yoga knowledge base? Do you need to do some more research, personal practice, study? Another option would be to bring in a yoga instructor to provide some detailed teaching or as a guest.

Yoga Camps

Kids love to go to camp, and yoga camp is no exception. Successful camps combine a variety of activities, engage children in active and passive rolls, provide opportunities for social development, and focus on both fine and gross motor skills. All of these pedagogical elements must, of course, be accompanied first and foremost by a spirit of fun and discovery.

At yoga camp, children are exposed to a more in-depth yoga experience than they would be at school or daycare. Discussions of *yamas* and *niyamas*, *pranayama* (breathing techniques), and meditation are easily introduced, and can be adapted to meet the needs and interests of each group. You may also be able to delve into areas that could be more suitable to this venue than a public school system setting.

Developing a daily theme based around one of the stories is a wonderful way to create a one-day camp. Fleshing out the curriculum with a story book, age-appropriate theme-based arts and crafts, songs, a healthy yoga-inspired snack, and yoga games will keep the pace lively and all participants having a wonderful experience. Remember that a child's attention span is roughly their age plus five minutes, so keep the activities changing and provide a wide variety of stimuli.

For a weeklong camp, pick a different theme for each day, being sure to include a variety of mediums for the craft projects. Revisit favourite games and activities throughout the week. Kids definitely love to have the teacher be 'It' during **Yoga Tag** (p.114), and **Swami Says** (p.114) becomes much more interesting and varied as the week progresses (more information on these activities can be found in **Chapter #7 Fun with Yoga)**(p.111). I have found that if possible, ending a summer camp with a no-holds-barred outdoor water fight is an ideal way to keep everyone laughing and having a great time.

A basic daily schedule will help the children know what to expect when. Parents also appreciate having a camp outline so they can prepare properly for camp, as well as discuss the daily activities with their child(ren). Starting with a gathering song will help the children to know when it is time to stop playing and sit in a circle to begin their day. Ending each camp session in a similar fashion provides a common thread, and completes the yoga experience.

Communicating clear expectations, maintaining a calm demeanour, and catching problems before they escalate are key elements in helping all children enjoy their camp experience. Instructors quickly learn who the group leaders are, and many discipline concerns can be alleviated by actively involving those individuals.

Yoga camps can be a childhood highlight if proper care and attention are put into planning and executing a rich and wonderful yoga experience. They provide an ideal setting with motivated participants, where all can explore the world of yoga while nurturing self-exploration and creativity.

Yoga for Special Needs

Before using yoga for anyone with special needs, please consult a physician or primary care giver. The activities and exercises here should complement—never replace—the advice of a licensed medical practitioner. Please follow the recommendation of certified professionals and continue to take any prescribed medications.

Sonia Sumar is considered the specialist when working with children with special needs. Her book, *Yoga for the Special Child*, and website, www.specialyoga.com, may prove especially helpful to parents, teachers, and caregivers who take care of children with these challenges.

ADHD

When diagnosing Attention Deficit Hyperactivity Disorder (ADHD), three symptoms are considered: inattention, hyperactivity, and impulsivity. Children with ADHD have one primary challenge: focus—whether lack of or fluctuations in focus, inability to refocus, or obsessive focus. Yoga *asanas* and breathing techniques can dramatically improve the ability to focus and can be used anytime, anywhere.

Students with ADHD who regularly engage in yoga are able to develop coping skills. Their self-esteem improves as disruptive behaviours are reduced. They are also better able to understand themselves and appreciate who they really are, and the contributions they can make.

Yogic practices of visualization, affirmations, and relaxation can prove especially powerful as behaviour therapy techniques. These can help increase attention span, improve the ability to relax, help regulate emotions, and teach stress-management skills. In addition, they will reduce stimulus overload by providing a sense of calm and inducing the relaxation response.

Partner and group poses further yoga's effectiveness in helping students with ADHD as they provide a forum for social skills training. The controlled environment with a short specific task, followed by positive reinforcement, is ideal for teaching the application of social skills.

Children with attention-deficit challenges benefit greatly from regular practice. Two to three times a week is optimal. Use pose cards such as *The Kids Yoga Deck: 50 Poses and Games* by Annie Buckley, or make your own using drawings or pictures of the poses in this book (a dog, a snake, a mountain, etc.). Children can then pick different groups of cards or poses for each session.

More information on how to assist students with ADHD can be found at the Canadian Attention Deficit Hyperactivity Disorder Resource Alliance (CADDRA) (visit www.caddra.ca) and the Centre for ADD/ADHD Advocacy, Canada (visit www.caddac.ca).

Autism

Children with Autism Spectrum Disorders will benefit from yoga since it addresses both the physical and emotional symptoms of the disorder.

The typical gross motor delay, hypotonia (low muscle tone), and impaired coordination of autism often result in low self-esteem and lack of confidence, which can extend to other areas of life. Yoga is an appropriate and enjoyable physical program which improves strength and tone in the muscles, develops balance, and increases body awareness. Even fine motor skills will be improved, as yoga emphasizes being in tune with the entire body, hands and fingers, feet and toes.

Children with autism may also suffer from sensory issues including sensitivity to light, noise, taste, texture, or smell. Furthermore, they may repeat movements that seem uncontrollable (self-stimulation behaviours). Yoga can help with these symptoms by soothing the nervous system and allowing pent-up energy to be released from the body in a non-competitive, peaceful manner.

The breathing techniques and guided visualization exercises also assist by reducing stress, teaching coping techniques, and providing a sense of calm and acceptance. Once a child has learned some of these exercises, they can use them anytime, anywhere.

When teaching yoga, take things slowly, introducing poses incrementally as comfort levels allow. Work on basic poses (**Mountain**, **Tree**, **Cat**, **Warrior**, etc.) and breathing exercises. Build one story at a time, gradually adding more poses.

To create visual stimulation and connections, line up stuffed animals or pictures of animals at the front of the room. Follow the line of animals, doing the pose for each in turn, creating an effective pattern. A similar exercise is to place the stuffed animals or pictures in a pile and have them picked at random, doing the corresponding pose each time.

A fantastic resource for teachers or parents wanting to use yoga for children with autism disorders is *Yoga for Children with Autism Spectrum Disorders* by Dion E. Betts. For further information regarding Autism Spectrum Disorders, visit the Autism Society of Canada on their website at www.autismsocietycanada.ca.

Cerebral Palsy

Cerebral Palsy is a group of injuries caused by damage to the brain and is the most common permanent disability of childhood. Compromised posture, tight muscles, and restrictive movement are characteristic of Cerebral Palsy. Yoga will help stretch and realign the spine, increase flexibility, and augment range of motion. Holding yoga poses in a gentle stretch helps relax the muscles, reducing high muscle tone, and exercising areas of low muscle tone.

Twisting poses are especially beneficial. A simple seated twist begins while sitting, rooting into the pelvis, inhale as you extend the spine/sit tall, exhale as you twist. Repeat two more times working deeper into the twist with each exhale. The last thing to rotate should be your neck with you gazing behind you. Release and return to centre. Repeat the process on the opposite side.

Standing poses (**Mountain**, **Compass**, **Warrior**, **Chair**), inversions (**Downward Dog**, **Dolphin**, **Rabbit**), and backbends (**Cobra**, **Dancer**, **Camel**) exercise the spine in many ways, lengthening the space between vertebrae and relaxing the pressure on nerves. As a result, nerve function is enhanced and muscle tension released, providing greater range of movement, increased coordination, and flexibility.

An exercise which is highly beneficial for children with cerebral palsy is to make a bolster out of a rolled-up blanket or large pillow. Have the child lie back on it with their arms resting by their sides. Gently roll and rock the bolster back and forth. This is a wonderful way to energize the spine and open the front of the body.

In addition, a focus on breathing exercises will increase spinal movement and strengthen stomach and back muscles while stimulating internal organs. Learning to use a complete breath will loosen muscles throughout the torso and increase respiratory control.

Chanting and using music will also provide needed stimulus and is most enjoyable. Often activities involving moving to music or sitting quietly and feeling the reverberations of *Aum* (p.4) are the ones which bring the greatest happiness and contentment as the connection with sound becomes more vital than any physical limitations.

More complete support can be found at the Cerebral Palsy Association of Alberta (visit http://www.cpalberta.com).

Down Syndrome

Down syndrome (DS) results from an extra chromosome added to an individual's genetic makeup. Yoga works on both physical and mental abilities for children with DS, and provides a personal physical therapy routine which can be practised alone or in group settings.

Hypotonia (or low muscle tone) is typical in most children with DS. Yoga will help strengthen the muscles, tighten the ligaments, and tone the overall body. Standing poses will be especially beneficial for instable knee caps, weak ankles, and flat feet. Twists, both active and passive, will assist in stimulating internal organs and provide relief from digestion issues and constipation.

Teachers should note, however, to watch that children do not overstretch while doing *asanas,* which may be a tendency due to the loose nature of their muscles and ligaments. Care should also be taken to modify poses when necessary to accommodate shorter limbs and smaller stature.

Breathing exercises and guided imagery focus on improving the central nervous system, and help develop body awareness, concentration, and memory. In addition, *pranayama* will help ease pulmonary hypertension and provide a safe physical workout for children with congenital heart defects often associated with DS.

Thyroid dysfunction is also common in children with DS, which will affect growth and metabolic rate. A regular yoga practice will help stimulate the thyroid gland, especially by practising **Shoulder Stand**. It is advised to learn this pose under the direction of a certified yoga instructor and to be certain that no atlantoaxial instability (instability where the neck connects to the spine) exists before doing so.

For further information, or to find a support group in your community, visit the Canadian Down Syndrome Society on their website at www.cdss.ca.

Chapter 3   The Stories

Stories tell us of what we already knew and forgot, and remind us of what we haven't yet imagined. — Anne Watson

The Stories

In my mind, yoga naturally flows into story form. The *asanas,* or poses, originally were inspired by the environment. When working with children, it makes sense to link **Crocodile**, **Boat**, **Pyramid**, and **Sphinx** poses (among others) to create an adventure in Egypt (see **Trip down the Nile**)(p.44). It also makes it really fun for the kids. Adding an environmental context to a yoga practice helps their young minds visualize the situation, the poses, the sights, sounds, and effects of the practice. The story format provides the setting for a personal journey and exploration of ourselves and the world. Furthermore, stories allow for a fluid yoga experience, with poses leading naturally from one to another, linked thematically, always with room for personal adaptation, addition, or deletion.

Adult yoga classes are generally quiet, serene, and focused. Poses follow a basic pattern of warming, working, and cooling with an infinite number of possibilities filling the practice time. Most adults are involved in a highly personal way with their practice, and are focused within, trying to follow the instructor's guidance, find their edge, open, engage, watch their alignment, and remember to breathe. This requires concentration, and there is usually not a lot of chitchat or rambunctious behaviour.

Children's classes—while following the same basic pattern of warming, working and cooling—are anything but quiet, rarely serene, and generally filled with wonder, exploration, laughter, spontaneity, and fun.

> **Life will go on as long as there is someone to sing, to dance, to tell stories, and to listen.**
> — Oren Lyons

The stories provided here will hopefully offer some guidance as to how to present, perform, and hold a 20-40 minute yoga session for children. They are not strict in their adherence to pose order, inclusion or exclusion. I often let the story unfold according to the children's imaginations and suggestions, borrowing and adapting *asanas* as we go along our journey. These are often

the most creative sessions, but do require a degree of familiarity with yoga *asanas* and the story format.

You will find the stories are very loosely written, and may feel choppy or lack cohesion when read alone. If you are a stickler for story-telling you may not even consider them stories at all, as they do not have a main character, conflict, or resolution. In that sense, they are more adventures or trips, which the class uses as a contextual framework for their yoga session. They provide the environment for interaction, learning, and discovery, which follows a general narrative.

If you are interested in storytelling in its pure form, you will want to visit www.storytimeyoga.com, where master storyteller and yoga instructor Sydney Solis has developed beautiful, morally rich stories based on cultural traditions from around the world.

Here, the stories have been developed to work with elementary school programs of studies for Kindergarten to Grade 6. Hopefully they will expand, integrate, and apply many of the concepts being taught in the classroom. Ideally, teachers will be able to open to a story which supports a current teaching theme and present it, one frame at a time, with little extra preparation.

The stories are written in comic strip format. Each story includes eleven poses. Only one need remain in order: the final *asana*, **Corpse** pose (*savasana*). Each frame includes a suggested narrative which incorporates one yoga pose that is shown in a photograph below the narrative. Feel free to add your own personal commentary. This is a framework within which creativity, interests, current events, and individual adaptations enrich the experience, increasing the social, physical, emotional, and intellectual understanding of all participants.

At the end of each narrative, show the class how to perform the pose, ideally leading by example, giving clear physical placement descriptions. Complete step-by-step instructions for each posture are included in **Chapter #4 Asanas** (p.67) which are most helpful for those who are not familiar with yoga *asanas*. Remember that children will not perform the poses perfectly. Basic guidelines should be followed and the intent of the *asana* kept in mind, rather than its ideal execution.

Also included with each story are music suggestions and literature options. These help to further the thematic understanding and engage more learning styles simultaneously. For example, **Sailing, Sailing** (p.40) is more interactive if you play the song 'Come Sail Away' by Styx, while imagining hitting the open seas on a square rigger. And the story book *Brown Bear, Brown Bear, What do you See?* by Bill Martin Jr. and Eric Carle, supports and reinforces the story **Mountain Magic** (p.38). In this way, the yoga experience becomes a cross-curricular learning endeavour, helping to enrich topics already in the classroom. See **Chapter #2 How to use Yoga** (p.7) for more information on how this can be accomplished.

Once you and your students are comfortable with the story format, feel free to take various yoga poses and create your own stories. A valuable language arts exercise is to give a pair or small group of students a few poses (e.g., **Mountain, Warrior, Rabbit, Wheel**) and have them create a story, then perform it for the rest of the class. They could also write it down or illustrate it to further their understanding, language development, or creative interests. The teacher could discuss many different aspects of story writing, including setting, mood, character development, or conflict.

I find that the stories naturally lead to discussions about:

- Geography: as we 'travel the world'
- Culture: showing sensitivity for the environment in which we reside
- Language: how do you say "hello" in Swahili?
- Animals: camels are the most interesting creatures!
- Anatomy: sitz bones ... where are they and why are they important
- Life lessons: balance poses teach us focus which helps us to learn balance in life off the yoga mat

I hope you will try all of the stories at least once before you find a favourite. I know I have mine, which I return to time and time again. Enjoy the journey, write your story.

You are the hero of your own story.
— Mary McCarthy

African Safari

Africa is full of excitement, adventure, and mystery. Let's go on a Safari and discover a corner of the Dark Continent.

Let's begin in a village filled with rondavels, unique thatch-roofed round homes made from sand and dung. The villagers greet us and show us to the **chair** (p.74) of honour, reserved for special guests. 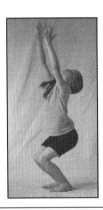	They are going to put on a show for us. First the **warriors** (p.99) come out. They are very fierce, strong, and brave. Look, they are carrying bows and arrows. Use your arms to shoot a bow and arrow. 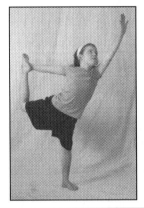	Next, the beautiful and graceful **dancers** (p.79) circle the fire. Balance first by focusing on a spot on the ground, then stretch. 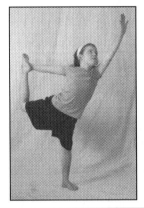
There are some very cute babies here in the village. **Happy baby pose** (p.84) is actually a very good hip opener. 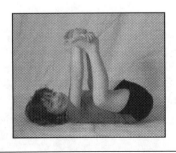	It's now time to head off on our adventure. There are lots of animals that graze across that savannah. Can you think of any? Zebras, wildebeest, gazelles, springbok, antelope are just a few. Let's do **deer pose** (p.79) to represent all these herbivores. 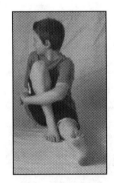	Let's keep going on our safari. We are so lucky! I see an **elephant** (p.82) in the brush. What sound does an elephant make? 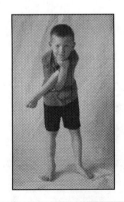

Oh my! Look carefully through the grass and you will see a beautiful **lion** (p.86). He is truly the king of beasts with his golden mane and mighty roar.

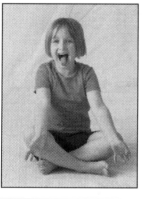

Now watch where you step as we go through this grass. There may be a slithering snake (**cobra pose**) (p.75).

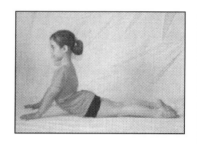

What a grand adventure! It's now time to clean up and take a shower at our hotel (**shower stretches**) (p.94).

You are true heroes of Africa. Let's do **hero pose** (p.85) and relax a bit after our adventure.

Now lie on your back (**corpse pose**) (p.77) and imagine watching a gorgeous African sunset. In your mind's eye, watch as the colours change from light blue, to dark blue, purple, pink, orange, gold, red.

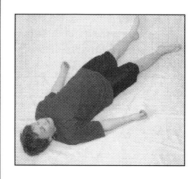

Literary Suggestions:

We All Went on Safari: A Counting Journey through Tanzania by Laurie Krebs, Barefoot Books, 2003

Water Hole Waiting by Jane Kurtz and Christopher Kurtz, Greenwillow, 2002

Music Suggestions:

'Africa' – Toto

'The Lion Sleeps Tonight' – Paul Simon

'The Elephant Song' – Eric Herman

Crawling and Flying

Today we're going to explore the world of crawling and flying creatures.

Most of these creatures live outdoors. As we become a **tree** (p.98), imagine all the life that your tree provides. Think about it as a place to live, protection from the elements, for food, or for oxygen. Trees are very important to the ecosystem.

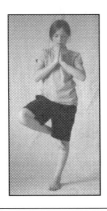

Another environmental contributor is a flower (**growing flower)** (p.83). There are so many different flowers, each helping beautify and enrich the world.

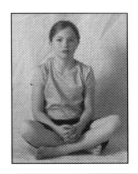

Often you'll find bees around flowers (**bumble bee lips**) (p.72). They are collecting nectar to take back to the hive where it will become honey.

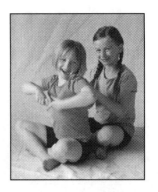

Another creature you may find in your garden, or out on the farm, is a grasshopper (**locust pose**) (p.87).

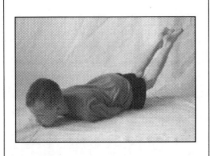

Another creepy crawly is an **inchworm** (p.85). They are actually moth larvae, and move by drawing the hind end forward while holding on with the front legs, then advancing the front section while holding on with the back legs. Give it a try.

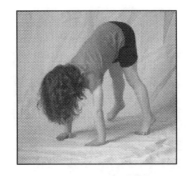

Arachnids (or spiders) also crawl, climb, spin, and sometimes float through the air (**spider**) (p.95). There are over 40,000 species of spiders which are found all around the world, except Antarctica. They have no antenna, eight legs, and fangs filled with venom.

One last crawling animal for today is the lizard (**crocodile pose**) (p.78). Lizards range in size from geckos to Komodo dragons. What type of lizard are you going to be today?

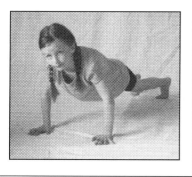

Now let's head for the sky. A common bird found in cities is a **pigeon** (p.90). Have you ever fed the pigeons in a park?

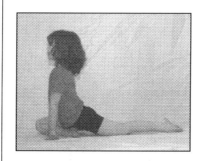

In the country you will see black crows. **Crows** (p.78) are highly intelligent but are often considered pests. They are sometimes used as symbols of doom or destruction in myths and stories.

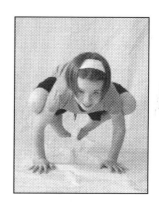

In contrast, **eagles** (p.81) are considered a sacred bird. Many First Nation peoples use eagle feathers in ceremonies and to honour leadership and bravery.

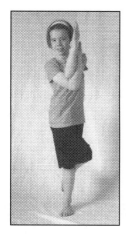

Now let's relax in **corpse pose** (p.77) by lying down, resting our hands by our hips, and closing our eyes. Inhale and exhale deeply and slowly, paying attention to each breath.

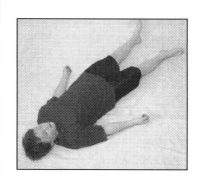

Literary Suggestions:

Sophie's Materpiece by Eileen Spinelli, Simon and Schuster, 2001

Music Suggestions:

'Eensy, Weensy Spider'

'Inchworm' – Danny Kaye

'Spider's Web' – Charlotte Diamond

Family Time

We all have a place to live and people who care about us.

Notice the corners of this room. They are made using right angles. Contractors build that way because it is very strong and can support the weight of the building. Let's do **mountain pose** (p.89). Your hips and shoulders are level and making right angles with your spine.

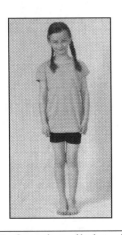

Around our home there are a few trees planted. Let's do **tree pose** (p.98) with our arms at shoulder height, perpendicular to our body. Imagine your toes are the roots, your standing leg the trunk.

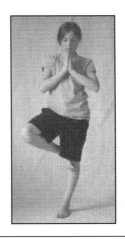

There may also be some tulips blooming in the front garden. Let's do **tiptoe pose** (p.97) and sing 'Tiptoe Through the Tulips.'

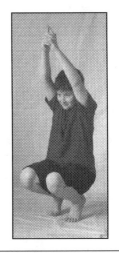

Look! I found a little girl's doll. **Ragdoll pose** (p.92) is very relaxing, as you let your body flop over just like a ragdoll.

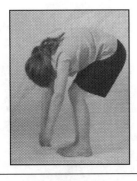

Ring, ring, ring. Sit down and grab your foot **phone** (p.90). Bring it up to your ear. Who are you talking to? Oh no, now the cell phone is ringing. Hang up and then hold onto your other foot.

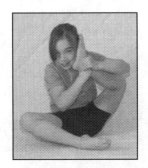

Now in our family we have a pet. **Downward dog pose** (p.81) is a really fun pose because you get to stretch just like a dog does when it wakes up. Be sure to wag your tail and give a little bark.

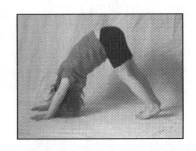

Maybe at your house you have a **cat** (p.73). They are so much fun as they pounce and play.

Oops, all that playing with the animals has woken up the baby. We need to **rock the baby** (p.93). That little tyke is getting a bit heavy so switch sides. Congratulations, you now have a very **happy baby** (p.84) in the house.

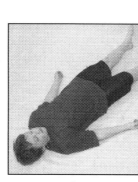

Since you made the baby happy, you get to have a treat. Let's try **two scoops** (p.99) of ice cream. You'll need a partner and let's make sure everyone knows how to do **child's pose** (p.74).

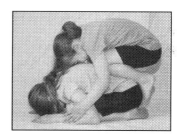

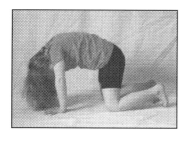

One last task before our day is done. We need to put some clothes into the **washing machine** (p.100).

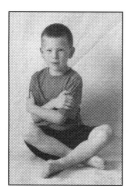

Now it's time to relax and enjoy being at home. Lie on your back (**corpse pose**) (p.77) and imagine taking a bubble bath. Allow your body to sink into the warm water and relax.

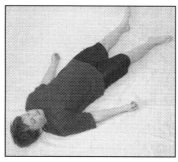

Literary Suggestions:

Hold My Hand: Five Stories of Love and Family by Charlotte Zolotow, Hyperion Books for Children, 2003

This is My Family by Gina and Mercer Mayer, Western Publishing Co., 1992

Music Suggestions:

'Why Did I Have to Have a Sister?' – Charlotte Diamond

'Skinnamarink'

Farmyard Fun

Today we are off to the Farm. How many of you have visited a farm before?

As we arrive, the dog comes out to greet us (**downward dog pose**) (p.81). He's a big ol' farm dog, friendly as can be. His tail wags in greeting.

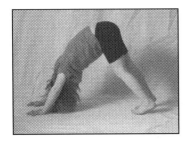

Next, we spy a barn **cat** (p.73), a very curious one of course, and great at catching mice. Be sure to meow and maybe even purr.

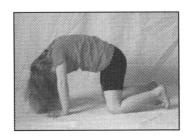

Off in the pasture we see a cow chewing her cud (**cow-faced pose**) (p.77). How can you tell if it is a beef or dairy cow?

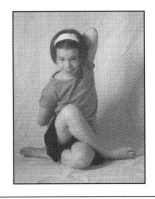

There is a **crow** (p.78) sitting on the fence post. Let's make the caw-caw-caw sound and bob our heads just like real crows.

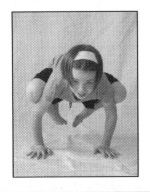

I see the Farmer's Wife has been very busy planting flowers and vegetables. Let's go explore her garden. First, we need to walk through the **gate** (p.83).

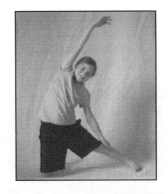

Oh no, they've had an unwanted visitor. A **rabbit** (p.92) has eaten lots of the vegetables. Pesky rabbits!

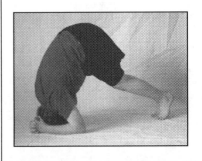

I see the Farmer off in the distance **ploughing** (p.91) a field. Everybody wave.

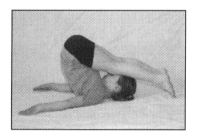

Today they use tractors and combines to do the work, but in the olden days they used oxen, cows, horses, or mules (**donkey kicks**) (p.80).

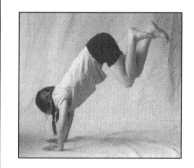

These animals often worked in teams and were harnessed together with a yoke to make them stronger, so we'll try a teamwork exercise (**back to back rises**) (p.70).

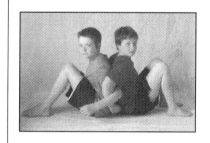

Once the harvest was in and the grain was taken to a mill, it was placed between two millstones, and a **wheel** (p.100) was turned to grind the grain into flour.

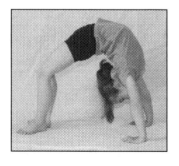

It's so much fun visiting the farm. Hug your knees up to your chest. Rock back and forth as if you were on a porch swing on the farm house veranda. Now lie on your back (**corpse pose**) (p.77). Imagine cuddling into a feather bed up in the guest room, cozy and warm.

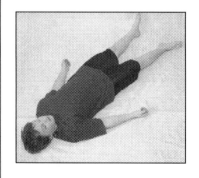

Literary Suggestions:

On Uncle John's Farm by Sally Fitz-Gibbon, Fitzhenrry and Whiteside, 2005

Wiggles by Christophe Loupy, North-South Book, 2004

Music Suggestions:

'Farmer in the Dell'

'Old MacDonald Had a Farm'

Garden Delights

Have you ever visited a Botanic Garden or someone's yard that is full of beautiful and interesting plants and flowers? Let's imagine going there today.

The first thing I notice are all kinds of flowers in the garden. We'll do two poses to represent flowers. First **lotus pose** (p.87). If full lotus is too difficult, stop at half lotus. Either one is a good stretch.

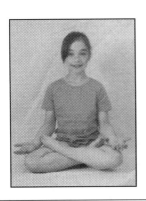

We can also tiptoe through the tulips with **tiptoe pose** (p.97).

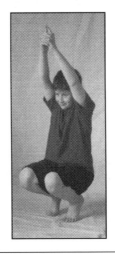

Did you know that there are some flowers that only bloom at night? Let's do **half moon pose** (p.84) so that we can enjoy these unique and wonderful plants.

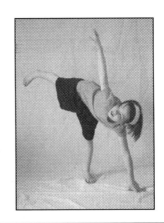

There are, of course, some bugs in our garden. I can see beautiful butterflies flitting from flower to flower (**cobbler's pose**) (p.75). Let your butterfly wings gently move up and down. What colour is your butterfly?

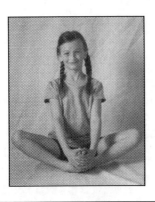

If you look closely, you may be able to find an **inchworm** (p.85). Let's see if you can cross the room while pretending to be inchworms. Focus on moving arms, then legs: one part of your body at a time.

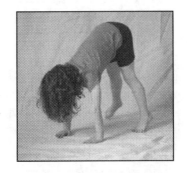

And there may be some bumble bees helping to pollinate the flowers as well. Let's make some bee lips that buzz (**bumble bee lips**) (p.72). Do you feel the vibrations in your throat, your face, and head? Doesn't that feel great?

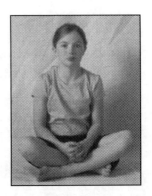

Over there I see a bird feeder. What kinds of birds do you see in your garden? I think today we will take the time to feed some **pigeons** (p.90). I love how they coo.

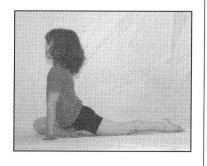

There are a group of children visiting the garden today on a field trip. Let's do **child's pose** (p.74).

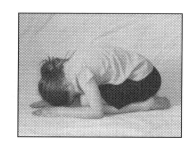

I see a water feature in the garden. There are large colourful koi in the pond. Let's do **fish pose** (p.82). Remember to make your fish lips.

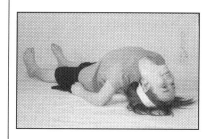

There is also a fountain with a water **wheel** (p.100) in it that turns. Long ago, water wheels were very important to grind wheat, but now they are simply decorative.

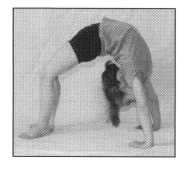

We've enjoyed a wonderful walk through the garden and have seen so many beautiful things. Now it's time to lie back on the cool grass (**corpse pose**) (p.77). Close your eyes and imagine looking up at the blue sky.

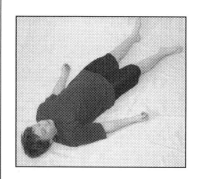

Literary Suggestions:

Who is in the Garden? by Vera Rosenberry, Holiday House, 2001

Good Morning, Garden, by Barbara Brenner, Northword, 2004

Music Suggestions:

'Tiptoe Through the Tulips'

'Each of Us is a Flower' – Charlotte Diamond

'Secret Garden' – Bruce Springstein

Man on the Moon

Today we are off on an adventure of a lifetime. We are headed to the moon! Have you ever wanted to be an astronaut?

Imagine that your hand is a star (**star (hand)**) (p.96). Make it shine dimly at first, then brighter and brighter. Now back off a little, choosing what level of intensity you want to shine at today. You are always giving off light, inspiring and guiding others.

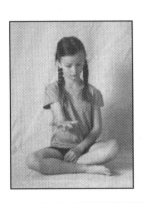

Before we can take off we need to do some **basic training** (p.70). One minute running in place, 10 sit-ups, 10 push-ups.

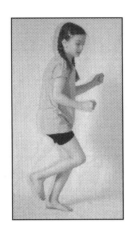

OK, now that we've passed the physical, we can become astronauts. Let's do **warrior pose** (p.99) and imagine being a brave astronaut preparing to go into outer space.

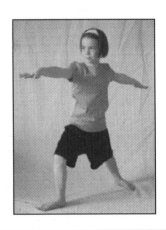

Now we need to make our bodies look like a **rocket** (p.94). Stretch your arms up overhead, intertwine your fingers, point your index fingers. Widen your legs, bend your knees and squat down. Countdown for lift off: 10, 9, 8, 7, 6, 5, 4, 3, 2, 1 ... Blastoff!

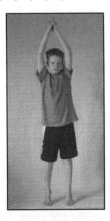

Now that we have left the earth's orbit, we have to work the controls to guide our space ship to the moon. **Compass pose** (p.76) will help us know which way to go.

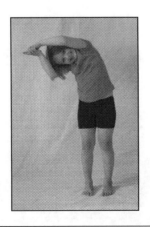

Look out the window. Do you see the moon? That's where we are going. Let's try **half moon pose** (p.84).

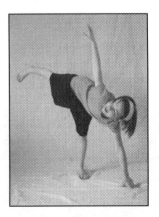

We're coming in for a landing. ten metres, five metres, two metres, one, touchdown. Perfect landing! Now we need to send the **robot** (p.93) out first. He will collect some samples and take pictures for research back on earth.

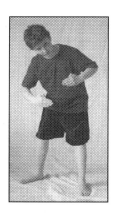

Now it's our turn. Imagine you are Neil Armstrong, who, in 1969, became the first man to walk on the moon's surface. As he stepped down he said, "That's one small step for man ... one giant leap for mankind." Let's all try to **moon walk** (p.89).

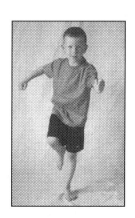

Hey, let's try out the **moon buggy** (p.88). You need to find a partner to sit with you. Now drive all over remembering that the moon has lots of craters: some small that feel like bumps on the road, some huge that you drive way down and then up the other side.

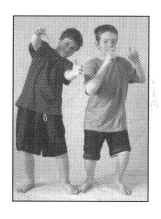

It's now time to return to the rocket and head back to earth. Let's lay on our backs and do a full body star stretch (**star (body)**) (p.96).

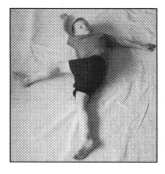

Now lay back and relax into **corpse pose** (p.77). Imagine you are floating in space, looking at the earth, seeing the blue oceans, white atmosphere, and green continents.

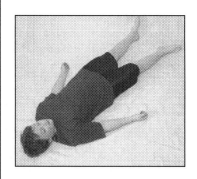

Literary Suggestions:

On the Moon by Anna Milbourne and Benji Davies, 2004

The Sea of Tranquility by Mark Haddon and Christian Birmingham, 1996

Music Suggestions:

'Twinkle, Twinkle Little Star'

'I Don't Want to Live on the Moon' – Shawn Colvin

Mountain Magic

We're off to do some camping in the mountains.

Everybody pile into the **bus** (p.72). Seat belts on! Stick together as we hit the open highway. 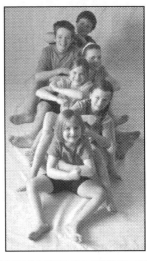	I can see the **mountains** (p.89). Mountain roads are really windy. Hold on around the corners. 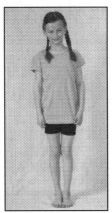	Hey look! A logging truck. Check out all those huge **trees** (p.98). Did you know that mountain air smells different from prairie air? Next time you visit the mountains, get out and take a deep breath to smell the air. It's fantastic! 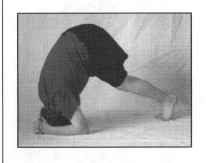
Let's go for a hike along this mountain trail. It leads to an alpine meadow. In the meadow we might find beautiful wildflowers (**lotus pose**) (p.87). 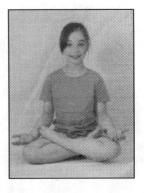	We also find butterflies (**cobbler's pose**) (p.75) floating from flower to flower. 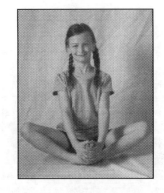	Quiet now, and stay very still and we'll see a brown **rabbit** (p.92) hop by. 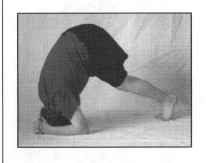

There are lots of different animals in the mountains. Can you think of any we might see along the way? Deer ... yes, all kinds of **deer** (p.79), elk, and moose live in the forests.

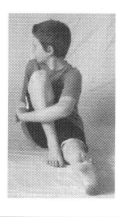

Bears ... Try a **bear walk** (p.71). Be sure to dig around for bugs, scratch your hips against a log (it's itchy on the other side, too), and rise up on your hind legs to growl as loud as you can.

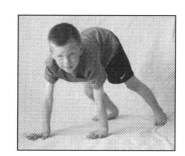

Eagles ... **Eagle pose** (p.81) is fun as you imagine holding firm to a branch and then getting ready to take flight ... 1, 2, 3 ... fly away!

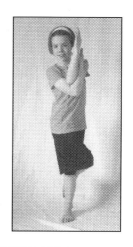
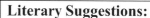

It's now time to make camp and set up our **tent** (p.97).

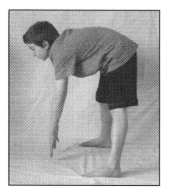

Lie on your back in **corpse pose** (p.77). Imagine a camp fire. Watch the flames as they dance in the darkness. It's toasty warm and people are telling stories and singing songs. Maybe you roast a marshmallow and taste its sugary sweetness as it melts in your mouth.

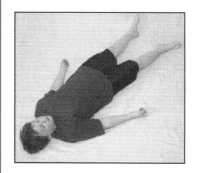

Literary Suggestions:

Brown Bear, Brown Bear, What Do You See? by Bill Martin Jr and Eric Carle, Henry Holt, 1967

The Tree in the Wood by Christopher Manson, North-South Books, 1993

We're Going on a Bear Hunt by Michael Rosen, Walker Books, 1989

Music Suggestions:

'The Bear Went Over the Mountain'

'Country Roads' – John Denver

Sailing, Sailing

It's time to go off on a grand adventure. All aboard! Today we get to be sailors!

First we board our square rigger sailing ship (**boat pose**) (p.71). Can you imagine sailing the seas on an old-fashioned wind-powered sailing ship? That would be so cool. 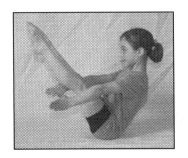	The captain of the ship was a fierce leader and **warrior** (p.99). He controlled the ship through strength, discipline, and loyalty. 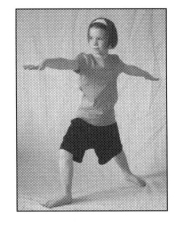	When on deck, the captain would take the helm or wheel and steer the ship. Let's do **wheel pose** (p.100) and try to make our bodies as round as possible. 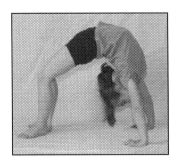
How would the captain know where to steer the ship? What would you use to know which way to go? The most ancient way to navigate your way across the sea is to use the sun, moon, and the stars (**half-moon pose**) (p.84). 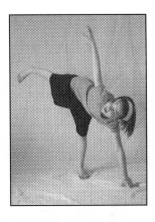	Next, we can try to make our bodies into beautiful shining stars (**star (body)**) (p.96). Do you know how to find the North Star or the Southern Cross? Constellations have always helped sailors to find direction. 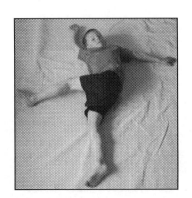	In more modern times, various navigational tools have been developed. The most common is a **compass** (p.76). 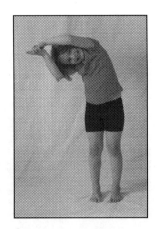

As we sail along, the **dolphins** (p.80) come out to play and swim along with the ship. Dolphins are highly intelligent, and are considered a sign of good luck for seamen. They are a symbol of joy, and you can imagine them leaping, playing and enjoying life.

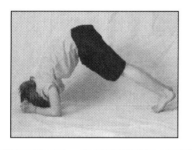

And here comes an albatross soaring on the trade winds (**eagle pose**) (p.81). There are all kinds of very interesting seabirds some of which fly great distances.

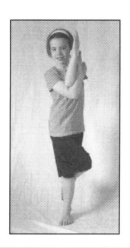

What do you think sailors ate while they were at sea for months at a time? I'm sure they brought as much food as they could, but I bet they also caught a lot of **fish** (p.82).

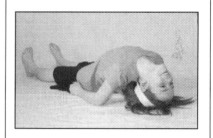

Hey, the kid up in the crow's nest is yelling something. Listen carefully, I think he sees land. What would you say if you saw land? "Land Ho!" That's right. There is a **mountain** (p.89) off in the distance, just coming over the horizon.

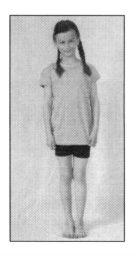

Yeah, we have completed our voyage. You guys were amazing sailors. Lie down and relax (**corpse pose**) (p.77) and imagine the ocean: deep, clear, endless seas.

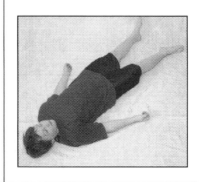

Literary Suggestions:

We're Sailing to Galapagos: a Week in the Pacific by Laurie Krebs, 2005

Dawn Watch by Jean I. Pendziwol, 2004

Music Suggestions:

'Come Sail Away' – Styx

'The Sailor Went to Sea'

Tour of India

India is such an interesting country. Let's go explore some of its great diversity.

Our first stop is a trip to the Ganges River. The Ganges is considered a holy river. However, it is not always a safe river. Long-snouted **crocodiles** (p.78) live within its waters.	There are also snapping **turtles** (p.98) which help to keep the Ganges clean.	Now, as we move along to visit the towns, we'll find many cows strolling about (**cow-faced pose**) (p.77). Cows are revered as a symbol of life and may not be killed.
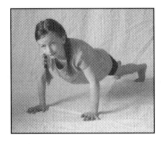	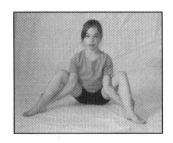	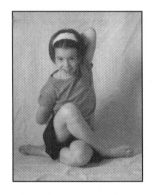
Now let's explore the north-western section of India. Here, we'll need a **camel** (p.73) to traverse the Thar Desert. Be sure to fill your hump with water, lifting your chest.	You may also find people living a traditional nomadic life. They live in **tents** (p.97) and move following trade routes, seasonal changes, and food sources.	India also has numerous National Parks, where we can explore the jungle. Of course, we'll see lots of **monkeys** (p.88) swinging from the trees.
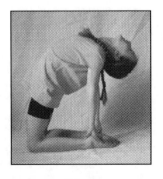	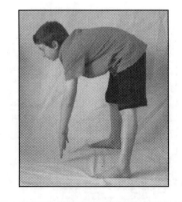	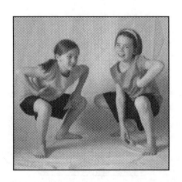

Be careful where you step, as there are over 270 species of snakes in India (**cobra pose**) (p.75). Remember to pull your shoulders away from your ears, making your neck lovely and long.

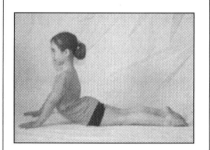

If we are very lucky while visiting the jungle, we'll glimpse a Bengal Tiger (**lion pose**) (p.86). There are only 1,800 Royal Bengal Tigers left in the wild, and they are considered an endangered species by the World Wildlife Foundation (WWF).

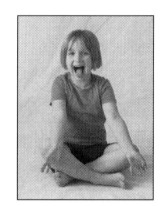

Finally, let's visit the Taj Mahal. It was built as a monument to love and reflects the beauty of the emperor's wife. Let's do **chair pose** (p.74) and imagine the empress sitting and enjoying the splendour.

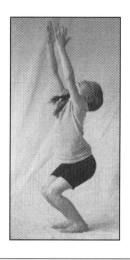

There may even be some peacocks strutting around the gardens of the Taj Mahal (**pigeon pose**) (p.90). Male peacocks, with their beautiful train and bright colours, are one of the most magnificent birds.

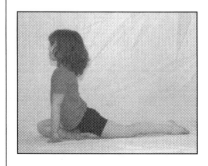

India truly is an incredibly diverse and fascinating country. You can now lie down on your back, hands by your hips, palms facing the sky (**corpse pose**) (p.77). Imagine riding in a hot air balloon looking down at the many places we just visited.

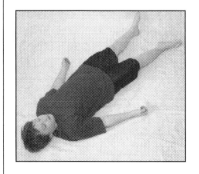

Literary Suggestions:

Once a Mouse by Marcia Brown, Aladdin, 1961

Nine Animals and the Well by James Rumford, Houghton Mifflin, 2003

Music Suggestions:

'Five Little Monkeys'

'Alice the Camel'

Trip Down the Nile

Let's go on an adventure down the Nile River in Egypt. What do you know about Egypt? Where is it?

Let's get into a **boat** (p.71) to begin our ride down the Nile. Did you know that the Nile is the longest river in the world, measuring 6,400 km in length? That's further than from Vancouver to Halifax.	What types of animals would you see along the Nile? **Crocodiles** (p.78) ... the Nile crocodile is one of the largest crocodiles in the world.	**Turtles** (p.98) ... the soft-shelled Nile turtle is huge and has cool yellow spots on its black back.
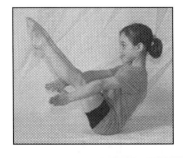	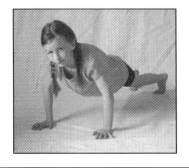	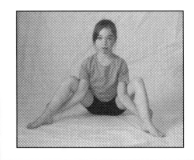
Now let's go for a **camel** (p.73) ride across the desert. What do you know about camels? Do you think it would be a smooth or bumpy ride?	Here is a beetle that was important to the ancient Egyptians. It's a scarab or dung beetle (**locust pose**) (p.87).	**Eagles** (p.81) and falcons are known throughout Arabia as being fantastic hunters. In fact, the earliest record of falconry is from Assyria, close to Egypt.
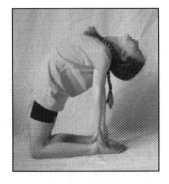	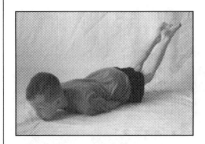	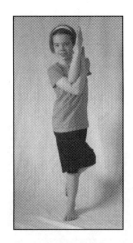

Exploring the desert is amazing. Imagine kilometres of sand in every direction. It's hot! It's dry! Oh look, I see palm **trees** (p.98) and water! It's an oasis!

Our camel has brought us to the Great Sphinx of Giza. A **sphinx** (p.95) has a lion's body with a human's face, and its role is temple guardian.

Let's visit the Great Pyramids of Egypt. The ancient pharaohs built amazing monuments. Try to be strong and immovable as you make a **pyramid** (p.91) with your body.

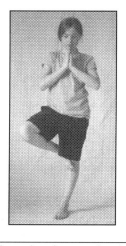

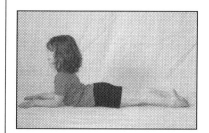

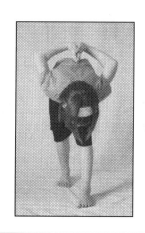

Which animal was buried in some of the tombs? **Cats!** (p.73) They have found hundreds of mummified cats which signifies great respect for these animals.

Now imagine that you are an Egyptian mummy, all wrapped up, snug and lying on your back. Close your eyes, relax (**corpse pose**) (p.77).

Literary Suggestions:

Skippyjon Jones in Mummy Trouble by Judy Schachner, Dutton, 2006

The Scarab's Secret by Nick Would, Francis Lincoln, 2006

Music Suggestions:

'Walk Like an Egyptian' – The Bangles

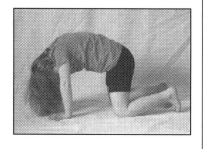

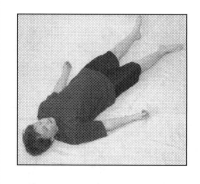

Amusons-nous à la ferme

Aujourd'hui nous irons à la ferme.

En arrivant à la ferme, un gros **chien** (p.81) sort pour nous accueillir. C'est un chien de ferme très amical. Sa queue remue sans arrêt pour nous montrer sa joie.	Nous remarquons ensuite un **chat** (p.73) de grange très curieux qui peut attraper toutes les souris. Assurez-vous de miauler et ronronner comme fait le chat.	Là-bas, dans le pâturage, nous voyons une **vache** (p.77) qui rumine l'herbe des champs. Pouvez-vous dire si c'est un bœuf ou une vache laitière?
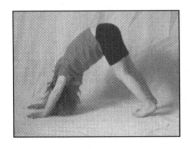	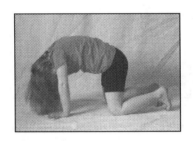	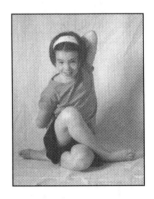
Sur le poteau de la barrière, un **corbeau** (p.78) se repose. Croassez et faites danser votre tête comme de vrais petits corbeaux.	Regardez! La fermière a été très occupée à planter des fleurs et des légumes dans son potager. Allons explorer son beau jardin en entrant par le **portail** (p.83).	Ôh zut! Ils ont eu un visiteur ravageur. Un **lapin** (p.92) a mangé un bon nombre de légumes. Quel lapin embêtant!
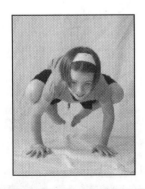	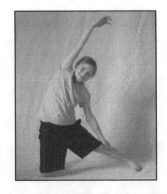	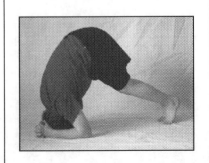

Je vois le fermier au loin labourant son champ (la **pose de la charrue**) (p.91). Saluez-le de la main.

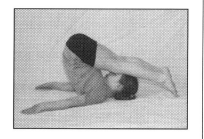

Aujourd'hui ils emploient des tracteurs et des moissonneuse-batteuse pour effectuer le travail, mais dans les temps anciens, ils employaient des bœufs, des vaches, des chevaux, ou des mules (**coup de sabots de l'âne**) (p.80) pour faire le travail.

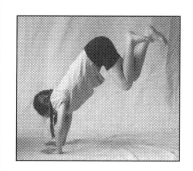

Ces animaux ont souvent travaillé en équipe. On les attelait avec un joug pour les rendre plus forts. Pareillement, nous essayerons un exercice de travail d'équipe (**élévations arrière dos-à-dos**) (p.70).

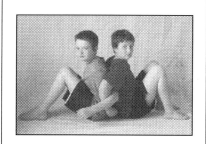

Une fois la moisson terminé, on amenait le grain au moulin. Le grain se fessait écraser entre deux meules qui tournaient grâce à une **roue** (p.100). Ainsi le grain était moulu pour en faire de la farine.

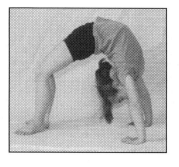

C'est très amusant de visiter la ferme. Serrez vos genoux à votre torse. Basculez-vous en avant et en arrière comme si vous étiez assis sur une chaise berçante sur la véranda de la maison de ferme. Maintenant allongez-vous sur le dos (la **pose du cadavre**) (p.77). Imaginez-vous dans la chambre d'invité blottis dans un lit de plumes confortable et chaud.

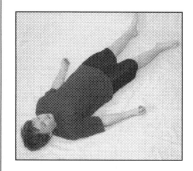

Suggestions littéraires :

Je découvre la ferme par J.M. Parramón, Bordas, 1989

Les Animaux de la Ferme par Karen Jacobsen, Children's Press Chicago, 1981

Chantons à la ferme par Bob King, Scholastic Canada, 1991

Suggestions musicales :

'Delvina la poule' – Carmen Campagne

'Mon père m'envoie au marche' – Carmen Campagne

'Vieux Mathieu a une Ferme'

Chez moi

Nous avons tous un endroit où vivre et des gens qui prennent soin de nous.

Vous voyez comme chaque coin de cette pièce est à angle droit. Les entrepreneurs construisent de cette manière parce qu'ils obtiennent une base solide pour soutenir le poids du bâtiment. Faisons la **pose de la montagne** (p.89). Vos hanches et vos épaules sont au niveau et forment des angles droits avec votre colonne vertébrale. 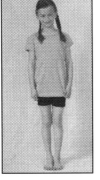	Autour de notre maison il y a quelques arbres plantés. Faisons la **pose de l'arbre** (p.98) avec nos mains que se retrouvent au niveau de nos épaules, perpendiculaire à notre corps. 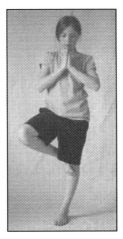	Il peut y avoir également quelques tulipes fleurissantes dans le jardin. Faisons la **pose de la pointe des pieds** (p.97). 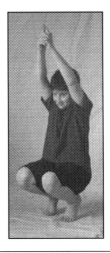
Regardez! J'ai trouvé la poupée d'une petite fille (la **pose de la poupée de chiffon**) (p.92). Permettez à votre corps d'être complètement détendu. Relâchez-vous et laissez votre corps effondre juste comme une poupée de chiffon. 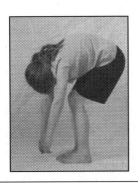	Dring, dring, dring! Asseyez-vous et saisissez votre **téléphone** de pied (p.90). Apportez-le jusqu'à votre oreille. À qui voulez-vous parler? Maintenant le téléphone cellulaire sonne. Raccrochez vite pour prendre l'appelle de votre autre pied. 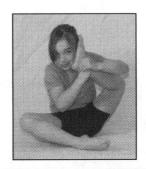	Dans notre famille nous avons un animal domestique. La **pose du chien à la baisse** (p.81) est une pose amusant parce que vous vous étirerez comme un chien le fait lorsqu' il se réveille. Assurez-vous bien de remuer la queue et de faire un aboiement. 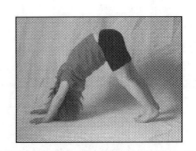

Peut-être bien que chez-vous, vous avez un **chat** (p.73). Il est tellement amusement car il sautille et joue sans arrêt.

Tous ces jeux ont réveillés le bébé. Nous devons **bercer l'enfant** (p.93). Ah! Cet enfant devient plus lourd; changeons de côté. Félicitations! Vous avez maintenant un **bébé très heureux** (p.84) dans la maison.

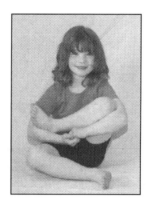

Puisque vous avez rendu le bébé heureux, on vous donne une gâterie. Essayons **deux boules de crème glacée** (p.99). Vous aurez besoin d'un ami et assurez-vous que chacun sait faire la **pose de l'enfant** (p.74).

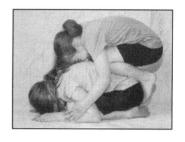

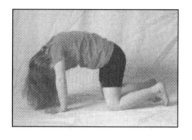

Il reste encore une corvée à accomplir avant de se reposer. Nous devons mettre quelques vêtements dans **la machine à laver** (p.100).

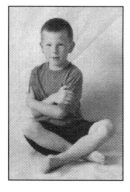

Maintenant il est temps de détendre et d'avoir plaisir à la maison. Allongez-vous sur le dos (la **pose du cadavre**) (p.77) et imaginez prendre un bain remplis de grosses bulles. Permettez à votre corps de descendre dans l'eau chaude et de se détendre.

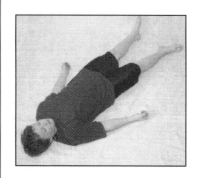

Suggestions littéraires:

L'alphabet de la famille, Fleurus, 2005

Dessine-Moi une Maison par Hélène Ray, Bordas, 1986

Suggestions musicales:

'Ma Famille Ma Parenté' – Alex Mahé

'Mille Façons' – Carmen Campagne

'Fais dodo' – Hannah Naiman

Hissez les voiles!

Il est temps de partir pour une grande aventure. Tous à bord! Aujourd'hui, nous serons des matelots!

Premièrement, montons à bord de notre bateau (la **pose du bateau**) (p.71). Pouvez-vous imaginer naviguer les mers sur un ancien navire à voiles poussé par un vent déchainé? Ce serait incroyable.

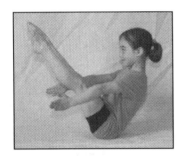

Le capitaine du bateau était un chef et un **guerrier** (p.99) féroce. Il commandait le bateau par la force, la discipline, et la fidélité.

Quand il était sur le pont, le capitaine prenait la barre ou la roue de gouvernail et dirigeait le navire. Faisons la **pose de la roue** (p.100) et essayons de rendre nos corps aussi ronds que possible.

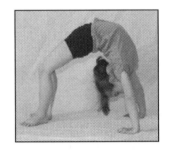

Comment faisait le capitaine pour diriger en bateau? Imaginez-vous ne pas avoir de repaire visuel comme la terre pour vous orienter. Que peut-t-on utiliser pour savoir dans quelle direction aller? La manière la plus ancienne de se diriger à travers la mer est d'employer le soleil, la lune, et les étoiles (la **pose de la demi-lune**) (p.84).

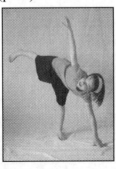

Maintenant, transformons-nous en une belle étoile brillante (**l'étoile (corps)**) (p.96). Savez-vous trouver l'étoile du nord ou la croix du sud? Les constellations ont toujours aidé aux marins à trouver leur direction.

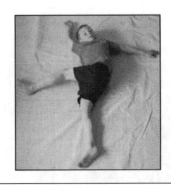

Aujourd'hui, de divers outils de navigation existent pour nous aider. Le plus commun de ceux-ci est la **boussole** (p.76).

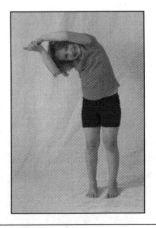

Tout en voguant sur la mer, les **dauphins** (p.80) nous rejoignent en nageant et jouant le long du bateau. Les dauphins sont extrêmement intelligents et sont considérés comme étant des porte-chance pour les marins. Ils sont un symbole de joie et vous pouvez les imaginer sauter, jouer et jouir de la vie.

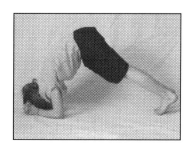

Un grand albatros vient nous rejoindre, planant sur les courants d'air chaud (la **pose de l'aigle**) (p.81). Il y a toutes sortes d'oiseaux marins qui volent de grandes distances.

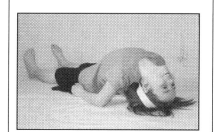

Que pensez-vous que les marins mangeaient tandis qu'ils étaient en mer pendant des mois? Je suis sûr qu'ils apportaient autant de nourriture que possible, mais je crois qu'ils pêchaient également beaucoup de **poissons** (p.82).

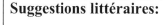

Hé, l'enfant perché dans la hune crie quelque chose. Écoute soigneusement, je pense qu'il voit de la terre. Que diriez-vous si vous voyiez de la terre? « Hohé, Terre! » C'est exact. Il y a une **montagne** (p.89) au loin se levant dans l'horizon.

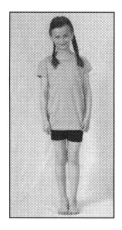

Hourra! Nous avons complété notre voyage. Vous étiez de super matelots. Couchez-vous et détendez-vous (la **pose du cadavre**) (p.77) et imaginez l'océan: profond, claire, de l'eau sans fin.

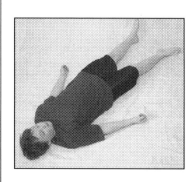

Suggestions littéraires:

Les bateaux par Daisy Keer, Éditions Épignes, 1996

Suggestions musicales:

'Une bateau mamie' – Hannah Naiman

'Partons la mer est belle' – 20 grandes chansons pour les ami(e)s

Le jardin joli

Avez-vous déjà visité un jardin botanique ou un jardin rempli de belles fleurs et de plantes intéressantes? Imaginons-nous en visiter un aujourd'hui.

Il y a toutes sortes de fleurs dans le jardin. Nous ferons deux poses pour représenter les fleurs. D'abord la **pose du lotus** (p.87). Si le lotus ouvert est trop difficile, faites le demi-lotus. Ce sera tout de même un bon étirement.	Nous pouvons également avancer sur la pointe des pieds par les tulipes avec la **pose de la pointe des pieds** (p.97).	Savez-vous qu'il y a quelques fleurs qui s'épanouissent seulement pendant la nuit? Faisons la **pose de la demi-lune** (p.84) de sorte que nous puissions apprécier ces plantes uniques et merveilleuses.
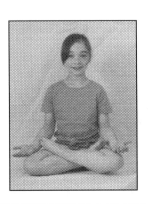	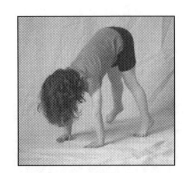	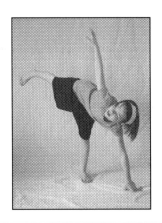
Il y a naturellement quelques insectes dans notre jardin. Je peux voir des beaux papillons qui volent d'une fleur à l'autre (la **pose du cordonnier**) (p.75). Laissez bougez vos ailes de papillon doucement de haut en bas. De quel couleur est votre papillon préféré?	Si vous cherchez bien, vous trouverez une **arpenteuse** (p.85). Voyons si vous pouvez traversez la salle tout en imitant une arpenteuse. Faites ramper votre corps en commençant avec les bras, puis les jambes. Bougez une partie de votre corps à la fois.	Il peut aussi y avoir des abeilles qui butinent de fleur en fleur (**lèvres d'abeille**) (p.72). Faisons le bruit d'une abeille qui bourdonne. Sentez-vous les vibrations dans votre gorge, votre visage, et votre tête? N'est-ce pas une sensation agréable?
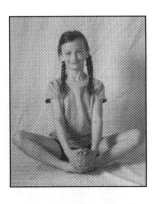	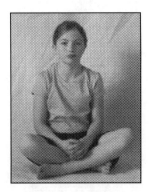	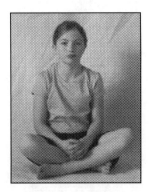

Là-bas je vois une mangeoire d'oiseau. Quels genres d'oiseaux voyez-vous dans votre jardin? Je pense qu'aujourd'hui nous prendrons le temps de nourrir quelques **pigeons** (p.90). J'aime bien leurs roucoulements.

Il y a des enfants qui rendent visite au jardin en excursion d'école. Faisons la **pose de l'enfant** (p.74).

Je vois qu'il y a un bel étang dans le jardin. Des grosses carpes colorées nagent dans l'eau. Faisons la **pose du poisson** (p.82). Faites bouger vos lèvres comme le font les poissons.

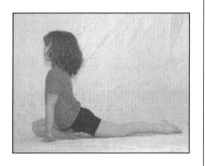

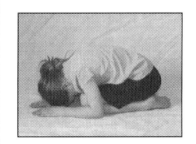

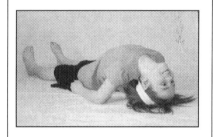

Il y a également une fontaine avec un moulin à eau (la **pose de la roue**) (p.100). Il y a bien longtemps les moulins à eau étaient très importants pour moudre le blé. Maintenant ils sont simplement décoratifs.

Quelle ravissante promenade nous avons faite dans le jardin. Nous avons vu tant de belles choses. Il est maintenant le temps de se coucher sur l'herbe fraîche (la **pose du cadavre**) (p.77). Fermez vos yeux et imaginez-vous regarder le ciel bleu.

Suggestions littéraires:

Dix petits grains par Ruth Brown, Gallimard Jeunesse 2001

Voilà mon jardin par J.M. Parramón, Bordas, 1988

Suggestions musicales:

'Nous sommes tous comme les fleurs' – Charlotte Diamond

'Savez-vous plantez des choux?' – Hannah Naiman

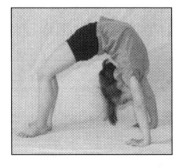

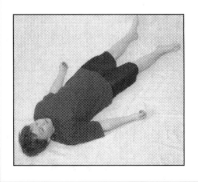

L'homme sur la lune

Aujourd'hui, partons pour l'aventure de notre vie. En direction pour la lune! N'avez-vous jamais voulu être un astronaute?

Imaginez-vous que votre main est une **étoile (la main)** (p.96). Au début, vous pouvez la faire luire faiblement, mais ensuite vous pouvez augmenter son éclat pour la rendre de plus en plus brillante. Permettez que peu de lumière se dégage pour l'instant, mais continuez à la faire briller. Rappelez-vous que vous dégagez toujours de la lumière autour de vous en inspirant et en guidant les autres.

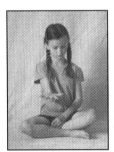

Avant que nous puissions partir pour la lune, nous devons faire une **formation de base** (p.70). Une minute de course sur place, 10 redressements assis et 10 pompes.

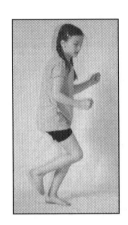

OK, puisque nous avons passé l'examen médical, nous pouvons devenir des astronautes. Prenons la **pose du guerrier** (p.99) et imaginons être un brave astronaute se préparant à entrer dans l'espace.

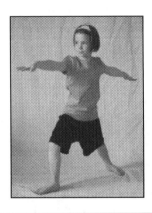

Maintenant nos corps doivent ressembler à une **fusée** (p.94). Étirez vos bras vers le haut, entre-croissez vos doigts en gardant vos index pointant vers le ciel. C'est bien. Écartez vos jambes, pliez vos genoux et accroupissez-vous vers le bas. Êtes-vous prêt? Le compte à rebours pour le lancement de la fusée commence: 10, 9, 8, 7, 6, 5, 4, 3, 2, 1 … Décollage!

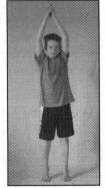

Maintenant que nous avons quitté l'orbite de la terre, nous devons garder notre vaisseau spatial en ligne directe pour atteindre la lune. La **pose de la boussole** (p.76) nous aidera à savoir dans quelle direction aller.

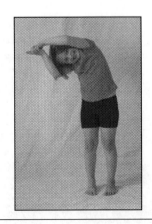

Regardez par la fenêtre, vous voyez la lune. C'est là où nous allons. Essayons la **pose de la demi-lune** (p.84).

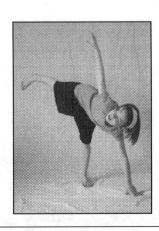

Nous nous apprêtons à atterrir. Dix mètres, cinq mètres, deux mètres, un mètre, enfin arrivé sur la lune. Atterrissage parfait. D'abord, nous devons envoyer le **robot** (p.93) à l'extérieur. Il rassemblera quelques échantillons et prendra des photos pour la recherche.

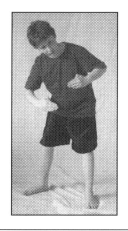

Imaginez que vous êtes Neil Armstrong qui, en 1969, est devenu le premier homme à marcher sur la lune. En posant son pied sur la lune, Neil a dit: « C'est un petit pas pour l'homme … un saut géant pour l'humanité. » Essayons la **promenade de la lune** (p.89).

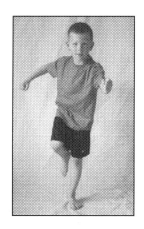

Embarquons dans le **véhicule lunaire** (p.88). Trouvez-vous un ami et assoyez-vous ensemble. Promenez-vous dans votre véhicule en vous rappelant que la lune a un bon nombre de cratères. Certains d'entre eux sont petits comme des bosses sur la route, et d'autres sont si creux qu'il faut que vous descendez lentement pour ensuite remonter cette côte raide.

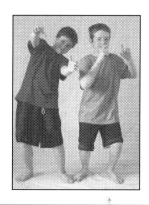

Il est maintenant temps de remonter dans la fusée pour repartir vers la terre. Étendons-nous sur le dos et faisons une **étoile** (p.96) avec notre corps.

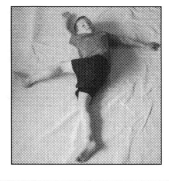

Maintenant remettez-vous sur le dos et détendez-vous complètement (**pose du cadavre**) (p.77). Imaginez-vous que vous flottez dans l'espace, regardant la terre, voyant les océans bleus, l'atmosphère blanche, et les continents verts.

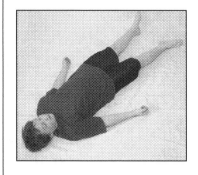

Suggestions littéraires:

La Lune par Paulette Bourgeois, Scholastic, 1996

Le Soleil, la Lune et les planètes par Stephanie Turnbull, Usborne, 2003

Suggestions musicales:

'Brille, Brille Petite Étoile'

'Au claire de la lune' – Carmen Campagne

'J't'aime gros comme le ciel' – Annie Brocoli

Les montagnes magiques

Aujourd'hui nous allons faire du camping dans les montagnes.

Embarquez dans l'**autobus** (p.72). Mettez vos ceintures de sécurité s'il vous plaît. Serrez-vous les coudes! On se met en route! 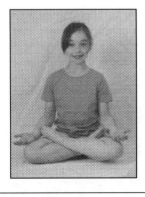	Je peux voir les **montagnes** (p.89). Les routes sont vraiment tortueuses. Cramponnez-vous pendant que l'autobus prend ce virage! 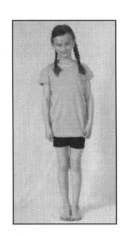	Regardez! Un camion pour bois tronçonnés. Les rondins sont énormes (la **pose de l'arbre**) (p.98). Savez-vous que l'odeur de l'air des montagnes est différente de celle des prairies? La prochaine fois que vous visitez les montagnes, prenez le temps de respirer à fond. C'est fantastique! 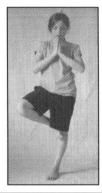
Venez! Nous allons faire une randonnée sur cette piste montagnarde qui nous mène à un pré plein de belles fleurs sauvages (la **pose du lotus**) (p.87). 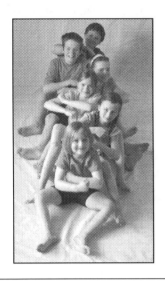	Il y a aussi des papillons (la **pose du cordonnier**) (p.75) qui volent de fleur à fleur. 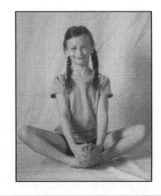	Si nous sommes silencieux et immobiles, peut-être nous aurons la chance de voir un **lapin** (p.92). 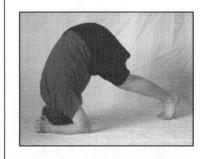

Il y a beaucoup d'animaux qui habitent les montagnes. On ne sait jamais quel animal se retrouvera sure notre chemin. Peut-être un **cerf** (p.79) croisera notre route. Il y a toutes sortes de cerfs, d'élans, et d'orignaux dans les forêts alpines.

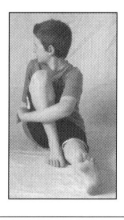

Les ours ... essayez de **marcher comme un ours** (p.71). N'oubliez pas de fouiller le sol afin de trouver des insectes. Frottez vos hanches contre un rondin. Mettez-vous debout sur vos pattes de derrière et grognez aussi fort qu'un grizzli.

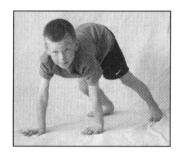

Les aigles ... La **pose de l'aigle** (p.81) est très amusante! Imaginez que vous êtes sur une branche, vos griffes percent l'écorce. Vous vous préparez pour le décollage ... 1, 2, 3 ... envolez-vous!

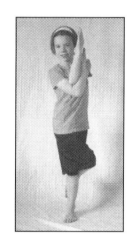

C'est le temps de s'arrêter et de préparer notre camp. N'oubliez pas de monter la **tente** (p.97).

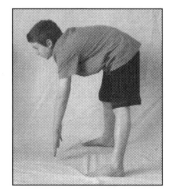

Allongez-vous (la **pose du cadavre**) (p.77). Imaginez un feu de camp. Regardez les flammes qui dansent dans l'obscurité. Le feu réchauffe les gens qui l'entourent. Écoutez les chantes et les histoires qui y sont racontées. Peut-être pourriez-vous faire griller une guimauve et savourez la texture pendant qu'elle fond dans votre bouche.

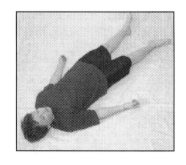

Suggestions littéraires:

Nos Forêts par Allan Fowler, Éditions Scholastic, 1999

La montagne par Maria Rius, Bordas, 1986

Suggestions musicales:

'L'arbre est dans ses Feuilles' – Alex Mahé

'Je suis prêt pour les montagnes' – Charlotte Diamond

'On fait du camping' – Matt

Ramper et voler

Aujourd'hui nous allons explorer le monde des créatures qui rampent et qui volent.

La plupart de ces créatures vivent à l'extérieur. Pendant que nous nous transformons en un **arbre** (p.98) imaginez tout ce que votre arbre apporte aux autres. Il est un refuge pour certains animaux, une protection contre les éléments pour plusieurs, de la nourriture pour d'autres, et simplement de l'oxygène pour tous. Les arbres sont très importants pour notre écosystème.

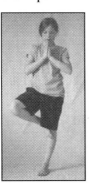

Un autre contribuant environnemental important est la fleur (**fleur croissante**) (p.83). Il y a tant de fleurs différentes, chacune d'elles embellissant et enrichissant la terre.

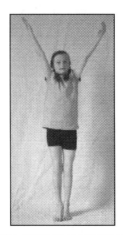

On retrouve très souvent des abeilles qui bourdonnent autour des fleurs (**les lèvres d'abeille**) (p.72). Elles récoltent le nectar pour ensuite le déposer dans leur ruche où il se transformera en miel.

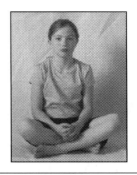

Un autre insecte que vous pouvez retrouver dans votre jardin ou dehors à la ferme est une **sauterelle** (p.87).

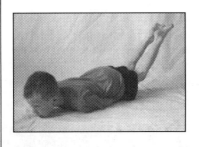

Une **arpenteuse** (p.85) est un autre insecte commun que l'on retrouve dans nos jardins. Celle-ci se déplace en approchant la partie arrière de son corps vers l'avant tout en se tenant sur place grâce à ses petites pattes de l'avant. Ensuite, elle pousse la partie avant de son corps le plus loin possible en se tenant sur ses pattes de derrières.

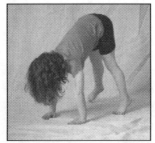

Les arachnides ou les araignées peuvent également rampent, grimper, et tourner (**araignée**) (p.95). Il y a plus de 40,000 espèces d'araignées que l'on retrouve dans le monde entier à l'exception, bien sûr, de l'Antarctique. Elles ont huit pattes et des crocs remplis de venin.

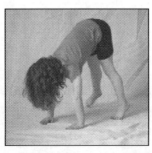

Imitons un dernier animal qui rampe. Préparez-vous à devenir un lézard (**pose du crocodile**) (p.78). Il existe des lézards de toutes tailles: dès les petits geckos jusqu'aux dragons des Komodos. Quel type de lézard allez-vous être aujourd'hui?

Maintenant dirigeons-nous vers le ciel. Le **pigeon** (p.90) est un oiseau commun retrouvé dans les villes. Avez-vous déjà nourrie des pigeons dans un parc?

À la campagne vous verrez des **corbeaux** noirs (p.78). Les corbeaux sont très intelligents mais sont souvent considérés comme étant des parasites pour la société. Ils sont utilisés dans les contes et les mythes comme symboles de malchance ou de destruction.

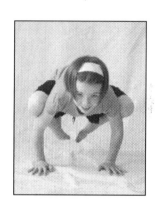

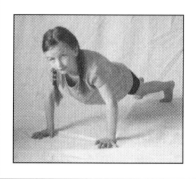

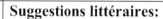

Par contre les **aigles** (p.81) sont considérés comme des oiseaux sacrés. Beaucoup de peuples des premières nations utilisaient des plumes d'aigle pour honorer ceux qui démontraient une conduite courageuse. Ils les employaient aussi pendant leurs cérémonies.

Maintenant détendons-nous et faisons la **pose du cadavre** (p.77) en se couchant sur le dos, laissant reposer nos mains près de nos hanches et en fermant nos yeux. Inspirez lentement et profondément puis expirez en prêtant l'attention à votre souffle.

Suggestions littéraires:

Le petit oiseau par Maria Rius, Bordas, 1986

Les insectes et autres petites bêtes par Amanda O'Neill, Les Éditions Héritage, 1995

Suggestions musicales:

'La toile d'araignée' – Charlotte Diamond

'Camille la chenille' – Carmen Campagne

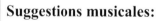

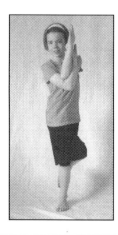

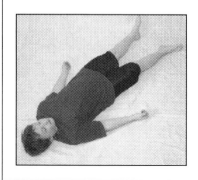

Un safari en Afrique

L'Afrique est remplie de mystères et d'aventures. Allons en safari pour découvrir un coin de ce continent phénoménal.

Commençons par une visite dans un village rempli de rondavels. Ces petites maisons uniques sont rondes et construites à partir de sable et de fumier. Un toit de chaume les couvre. Les villageois nous saluent et nous invitent à prendre place sur la **chaise** (p.74) d'honneur, réservée pour les invités spéciaux.

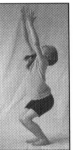

Ils nous ont préparé un spectacle. D'abord les **guerriers** (p.99) sortent. Ils sont très féroces, courageux et forts. Regardes, ils portent des arcs et des flèches. Tirez une flèche avec vos bras.

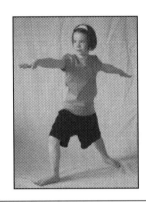

Ensuite, les beaux **danseurs** (p.79) remplie de grâce font la ronde autour du feu. Gardez votre équilibre en fixant un point sur le plancher, puis étirez-vous bien.

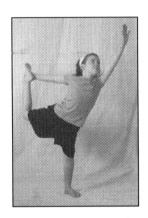

Dans le village il y a quelques bébés très mignons et bien potelés. La **pose de l'enfant heureux** (p.84) rendra vos hanches souples.

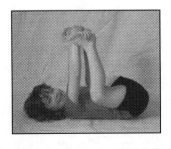

Maintenant c'est l'heure de commencer notre aventure. Regardez là-bas! Il y a plusieurs animaux qui broutent dans la savane. Lesquels voyez-vous? Il y a des zèbres, des gazelles, des springboks, des antilopes, des gnous, pour en nommer quelques-uns. Faisons la **pose du cerf** (p.79) pour représenter tous ces herbivores.

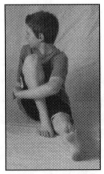

Continuons notre safari. Nous sommes si chanceux. Je vois un **éléphant** (p.82) là, dans la brousse. Quel bruit fait les éléphants?

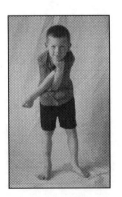

Regardez soigneusement à travers les hautes herbes et vous verrez un beau **lion** (p.86). Il est vraiment le roi des animaux avec sa crinière d'or et son hurlement puissant.

Faîtes attention tout en marchant dans les hautes herbes de ne pas marcher accidentellement sur un serpent (**pose du cobra**) (p.75).

Quelle grande aventure. Il est maintenant l'heure de se laver en prenant une bonne douche à notre hôtel. (les **étirements de la douche**) (p.94).

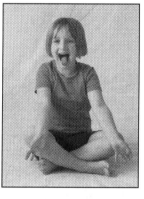

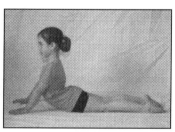

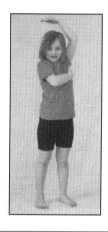

Vous êtes les vrais héros de l'Afrique. Détendons-nous dans la **pose du héros** (p.85).

Maintenant nous pouvons nous allonger sur le dos (**pose du cadavre**) (p.77) et imaginer un magnifique coucher du soleil africain. Dans votre esprit, remarquez les couleurs, qui changent de bleu-clair à bleu-foncé, puis à rose, orange, or, rouge, et finalement en violet,

Suggestions littéraires:

Comment les girafes dissent-elles maman? par Willi Glasauer, L'école des loisirs, 2004

Croque, le crocodile par Josephine Croser, Scholastic, 1986

Suggestions musicales:

'Mustafa' – Carmen Campagne

'Cedo: Celebration Songs for Children' – Louise Raymond

'Un éléphant se balançait'

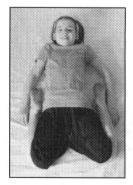

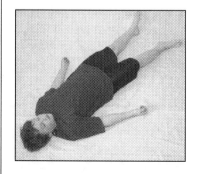

Un tour en Inde

L'Inde est un pays fascinant! Allons explorer une partie de sa grande diversité.

D'abord nous explorons le Gange. Le Gange est considéré comme un fleuve sacré. Cependant, ce n'est pas toujours un fleuve sans danger. Les **crocodiles** Gavial du Gange (p.78) vivent dans ces eaux.	Nous trouverons également des **tortues** (p.98) dans le Gange. Elles aident à garder le fleuve propre.	Tout en descendant le long du fleuve, nous croisons de nombreux petits villages et bien sûr, nous voyons plusieurs **vaches** (p.77). Elles sont vénérées parce qu'elles représentent et symbolisent la vie. On ne les tues jamais.
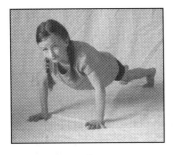	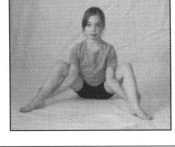	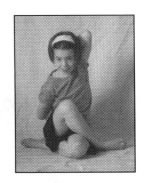
Parcourons maintenant la section occidentale du nord de l'Inde. Ici, nous aurons besoin d'un **chameau** (p.73) pour traverser le désert de Thar. Soyez sûr de remplir votre bosse avec de l'eau, soulevant bien votre poitrine.	Vous pouvez également trouver des personnes vivant une vie traditionnelle de nomade. Ils vivent dans des **tentes** (p.97) et suivent les routes de commerce, les changements saisonniers, et les sources de nourriture.	L'Inde a également un bon nombre de parcs nationaux, où nous pouvons explorer la jungle. Naturellement, nous verrons plein de **singes** (p.88) se balançant dans les arbres.
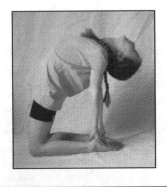	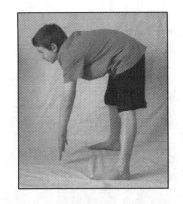	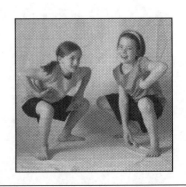

Faites attention où vous marchez! Il y a plus de 270 espèces de serpents en Inde (la **pose du cobra**) (p.75). Rappelez-vous de tirer les épaules loin des oreilles, rendant votre cou beau long.

Si nous sommes chanceux, nous apercevrons peut-être un tigre royal du Bengale (la **pose du lion**) (p.86) dans cette belle jungle que nous visitons. Il ne reste que 1,800 tigres du Bengale en liberté et ils sont considérés une espèce en voie de disparition par le WWF.

Enfin, visitons le Taj Mahal. Il a été construit comme monument reflétant l'amour et la beauté de l'épouse de l'empereur. Faisons la **pose de la chaise** (p.74) et contemplons la reine qui a inspiré tout cette beauté.

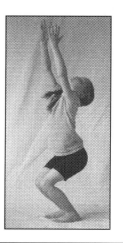

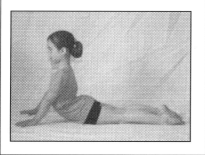

Il peut même y avoir quelques paons se pavanant autour des jardins du Taj Mahal (la **pose du pigeon**) (p.90). Les paons mâles exposent fièrement leur magnifique plumage multicolore. Ils sont réellement l'un des plus magnifiques oiseaux du monde.

L'Inde est un pays incroyablement divers et fascinant. Vous pouvez maintenant vous couchez sur le dos, les mains près de vos hanches, paumes faisant face au ciel (la **pose du cadavre**) (p.77). Imaginez monter dans une montgolfière, regardant tous les endroits que nous venons de visiter.

Suggestions littéraires:

Aujourd'hui en Inde par Patrice Favaro, Éditions Gallimard Jeunesse, 2005

Inde par Elaine Jackson, QED Publishing 2004

Suggestions musicales:

'Jai Ho' – A.R. Rahman

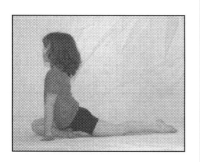

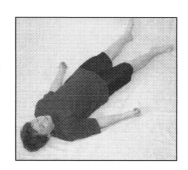

Une voyage sur la rivière Nil

Partons en aventure en voguant sur la rivière du Nil en Égypte. Que connaissez-vous de l'Égypte?

Embarquons dans un **bateau** (p.71) pour naviguez sur le Nil. Saviez-vous que le Nil est le plus long fleuve au monde mesurant 6.400 kilomètres de longueur? Il est aussi long que la distance entre Vancouver et Halifax.	Quels types d'animaux verriez-vous le long du Nil? Des **crocodiles** (p.78) … les crocodiles du Nil sont parmi les plus grands crocodiles au monde.	Des **tortues** (p.98) … les tortues molles du Nil sont énormes et ont des taches jaunes sur leur carapace noire.
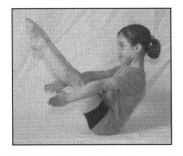	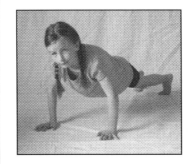	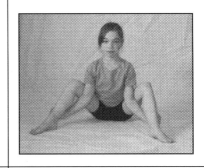
Traversons maintenant un désert sur le dos d'un **chameau** (p.73). Que connaissez-vous des chameaux? Est-ce que notre promenade sur leur dos sera reposante ou agitée?	Voici un coléoptère qui était important pour les Égyptiens d'autre-temps. C'est un scarabée ou un bousier (la **pose de la locuste**) (p.87).	Les **aigles** (p.81) et les faucons sont connus par l'Arabie comme étant des chasseurs fantastiques. La fauconnerie semble trouver son origine en Assyrie qui se situe tout près de l'Égypte.
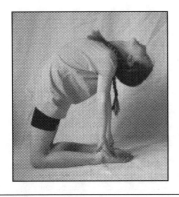	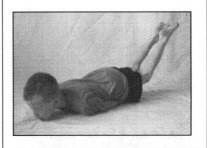	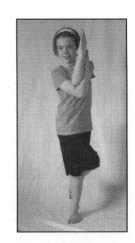

Explorer le désert est extraordinaire. Imaginez des kilomètres et des kilomètres de sable dans toutes les directions. Il fait chaud! C'est sec! Oh, regardez! Je vois des palmiers, de l'eau! C'est une oasis! (la **pose de l'arbre**) (p.98)

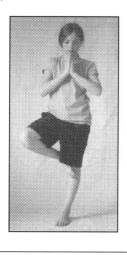

Notre chameau nous a emportés près du grand sphinx de Gizeh. Un **sphinx** (p.95) a un corps de lion avec une tête humaine. Il est le gardien du temple.

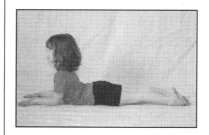

Allons visiter les grandes pyramides d'Égypte. Les pharaons d'autrefois ont construit ces monuments majestueux. Essayez d'être fort et immobile lorsque vous faites une **pyramide** (p.91) avec votre corps.

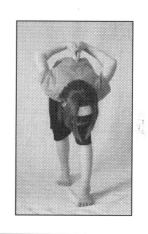

Quel animal était enterré dans certains tombeaux? Des **chats**! (p.73) Ils ont trouvé des centaines de chats momifiés, ce qui signifie que les égyptiens avaient un grand respect pour les chats.

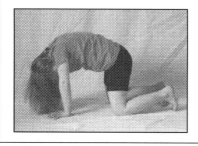

Maintenant, imaginez-vous que vous êtes une momie égyptienne, toute enveloppée et couchée confortablement sur votre dos. Fermez vos yeux et détendez-vous (la **pose du cadavre**) (p.77).

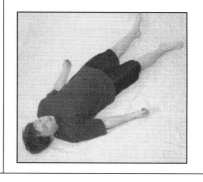

Suggestions littéraires:

Égypte par Elaine Jackson, QED Publishing, 2004

Suggestions musicales:

Petite Enfant (berceuse égyptienne) – dodo la planète do

'Sur la Bosse à Nova' – Shilvi

Chapter 4   Asanas

I'm carried on my breath like a leaf on the wind: folding, arching, twisting, bending, leaping lightly from one posture to the next. My body tingles with energy; my mind is quietly absorbed in the hypnotic rhythm of practice. — Anne Cushman

Basics of Asana Practice

The physical practice of yoga is founded upon numerous *asanas* referred to as poses or postures in English. Originally *asanas* served as stable postures for prolonged meditation. They have developed into an extensive repertoire of physical poses which help balance and tone the entire body. Each *asana* incorporates various parts and functions of the body, including the muscles, metabolism, circulation, hormones, and internal organs. They purify and strengthen the body, and focus the mind.

Contrary to popular perception, *asana* practice is not about how flexible or strong you are. It is about paying attention to how your body feels, how it moves, and about respecting who you are today while working to improve yourself for tomorrow.

Any *asana* has one of these common positions as a starting point:

Standing: supported on the soles of the feet

Sitting: supported on the base of the pelvis

Kneeling: supported on the knees, shins, and tops of feet

Supine: supported on the back surface of the body

Prone: supported on the front surface of the body

In addition to the starting point, the base of support for each *asana* must also be considered. This refers to the parts of the body which come in contact with the earth, and on which the weight will rest. Standing poses, which use the anatomically efficient feet, legs and pelvis to support the body's weight, are generally considered the foundation of *asana* practice (e.g., **Mountain**, **Warrior**). Arm-support poses, which employ the hands and arms to support weight, are structurally disadvantaged, and are considered intermediate or advanced (e.g., **Crocodile**, **Crow**).

Asanas are further divided into sections, depending on the movement created:

Forward bend: bending in a forward motion, from the hips, lengthening the back body

Back bend: bending backward, opening the front body

Twist: a twisting movement of the spine

Lateral bend: bending to one side, feeling the stretch in the side body

Some basic principles which assist with a safe and productive *asana* practice include:

Keep Breathing

Without the breath there is no life. Breathe slowly and deeply, in and out through the nose. You can direct your breath into areas of tension, but most children cannot do this until they develop greater body awareness and maturity. More detailed breathing exercises and descriptions are found in **Chapter 5 Breathing** (p.101).

> **Basic breathing guidelines for *asana* practice include:**
>
> **Inhale** as you expand, lift or open your body.
>
> **Exhale** as you contract or close your body.

Be Aware of Balance

In order to achieve balance equal amounts of effort and relaxation are key. In yogic terms, this is referred to as the polarities *sukha* (easy, pleasant, gentle) and *sthira* (solid, durable, strong). The ability to relax various muscles while working others requires effort and concentration.

Use Your Energy

Harness life's energy. Radiate from your core, outward, engaging your vital energy to create a body and mind that are strong but flexible. Remember to always work within a safe energy level, accepting what the body is able to do and the gift that it is. A great *asana* to teach this concept is **Star (hand)**(p.96).

Watch Your Alignment

Aim for straight lines and right angles. For example, when creating a **Table**, place hands below the shoulders, knees below the

> **These two simple verbal prompts will help students self correct their alignment**
>
> **Shoulder check: shoulders should be level and pulled away from the ears, creating strength and length (e.g. Mountain, Cobra)**
>
> **Knee check: if the leg is straight, knees are lifted with quadriceps engaged (e.g., Mountain); if the leg is bent, the knee should be directly over the ankle, with the ankle forming a 90-degree angle (e.g., Warrior)**

hips. The definitive guide on yoga alignment is *Light on Yoga* by B.K.S. Iyengar.

Pay Attention

Keep your eyes open, and your mind aware of your body and breath. Focus is essential. Pay attention to what you are doing and how it feels. Stretches should not be painful, but should ask your body to use and strengthen areas of weakness, while relaxing and loosening areas of tension. Center your attention by finding a focal point. This is especially useful in balance postures (e.g., **Eagle**, **Dancer**), and teaches concentration and focus. As children become more adept, you can explore various *drishti,* which are focus-points used with *asanas* or meditation.

Opposite Forces Attract

The elemental concept of push/pull is central to yogic thought and practice. When performing *asana*, push into the ground while extending up. Suction the muscles to the bones but relax and find space within. Try to remember the image of a rope with the fibres being wound in opposite directions. In standing poses, you push your big toe into the ground while the hip rotates out and back, creating a solid foundation (e.g., **Pyramid**). The same is true with the arms in **Downward Dog**, as the base of the thumb, index, and middle fingers are actively pressed into the floor, while the upper arms rotate outward and the shoulder blades pull down toward the tailbone.

These points are fairly advanced concepts and are not expected to be perfected in children. I've included them here to give adults a thorough understanding of *asanas* and to promote a safe and correct practice.

Back to Back Rises – Élévations arrière dos-à-dos

- With a partner who is of a similar size, sit back to back
- Intertwine arms
- Try to stand up without letting go of one another by working together, using your legs to push against your partner—this is harder than it first appears
- Try to sit down again

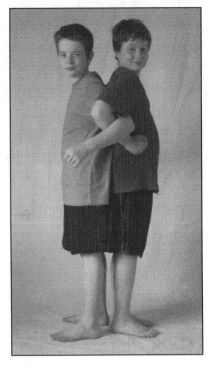

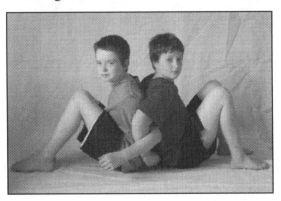

Basic Training – La formation de base

- Run on the spot; start slow then increase the pace; knees high; back kicks; sprint
- Sit-ups—as many as you are old
- Push-ups—as many as you are old

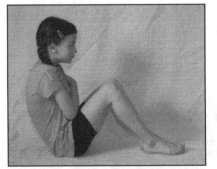

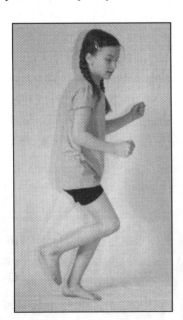

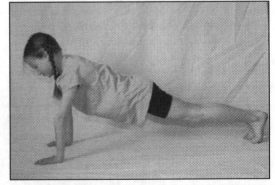

Bear Walk – Marcher comme un ours

- Stand, feet slightly apart
- Bend forward, placing your hands flat on the floor, knees slightly bent
- Imitate a bear by walking slowly like a large bear, left leg first, then left arm, followed by right leg, then right arm. Continue in this fashion. Try to run, dig for insects, crawl into a log, stand on your hind legs and roar

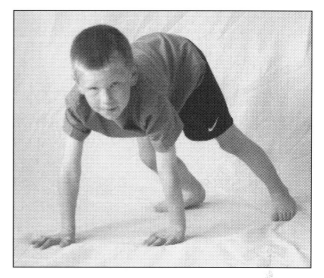

Boat – Le bateau

(Navasana)

- Sit, feet stretched out on the floor in front of you
- Bend your knees, placing the hands under the legs to hold on
- Keeping your back straight, shoulder blades pulled down, lift your feet off the floor
- If this is easy, release the hands, holding them parallel to the floor
- If this is easy, try to straighten your legs without rolling back onto your tailbone

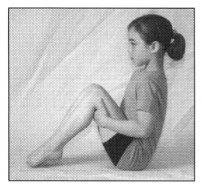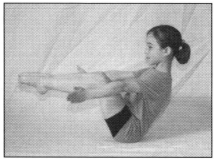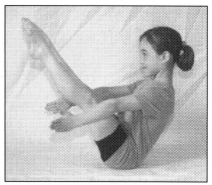

Bumble Bee Lips – Les lèvres d'abeille

- Sit cross-legged
- Inhale fully through your nose
- Exhale through the nose and make a rounded, steady humming 'mmmm' sound
- Listen to the sound, vary its pitch, move it around in your head and chest until you find a hum that feels comfortable and makes the lips buzz
- Repeat for 5-10 breaths, trying to maintain the hum for as long as possible each time

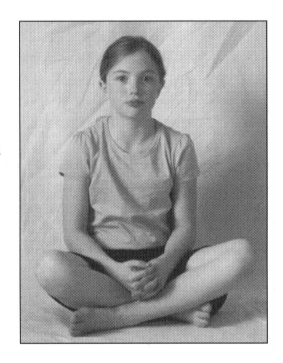

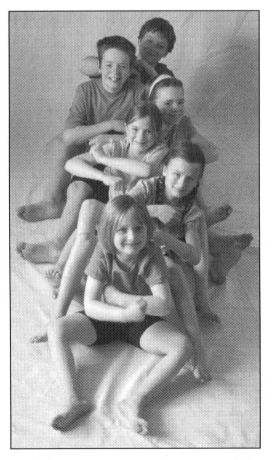

Bus – L'autobus

- Sit in a row behind one another, legs out to the sides of the person in front
- Roll your hands like the wheels of the bus
- Sing 'The Wheels on the Bus' as you scoot forward on your bottoms in unison
- Return to your mats

Camel – Le chameau

(Ustrasana)

- Kneel tall, tops of feet flat on the ground or toes curled under, whichever is most comfortable
- Circle one arm overhead, then reach for the heel behind you
- Circle the other arm, reaching for the other heel
- Lift your chest, filling the camel's hump with water
- If comfortable, allow your head to fall back

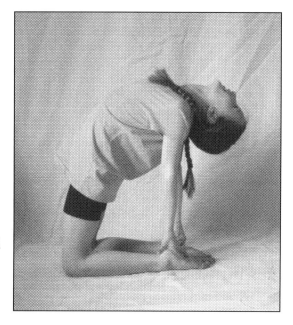

Cat – Le chat

(Marjarasana)

- Kneel on all fours in **Table** position
- Look up to the ceiling, allowing your back to sway, hips high, shoulders blades pulled down
- Round in the opposite direction, looking at your navel
- Repeat, inhaling as you look up, exhaling when looking down
- Stretch your back as much as possible in both directions

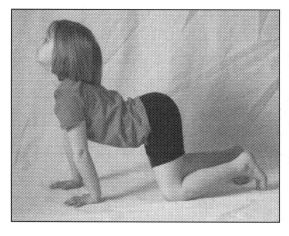
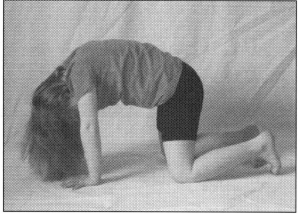

Chair – La chaise
(Utkatasana)

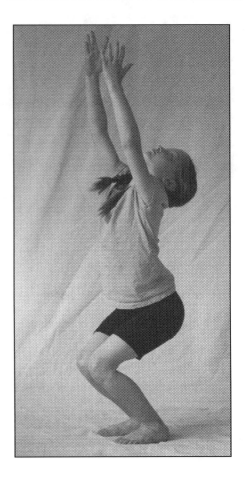

- Stand, feet together
- Inhale as you bend your knees and raise your hands over head, keeping your shoulder blades pulled down
- Hold for a few deep breaths

Child's Pose – L'enfant
(Balasana)

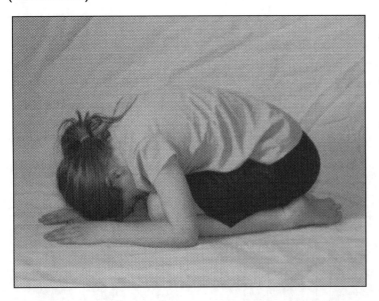

- Kneel low, rest your head on the floor in front of you
- Place your hands wherever it is comfortable
- Relax and breathe

Cobbler's Pose – Le cordonnier

(Baddha konasana)

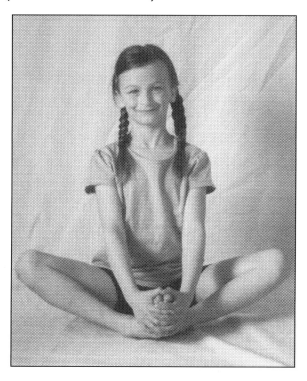

- Sit, bend your knees, and bring the soles of your feet together in front of you
- Allow your knees to open while sitting tall
- Gently raise and lower your knees slightly like a butterfly's wings

Cobra – Le cobra

(Bhujangasana)

- Lie on your stomach with your hands below your shoulders
- Inhale and slowly come up, lifting the head and torso, keeping the elbows touching the ribs and shoulder blades pulled down
- Exhale and return to the floor, chin leading
- Repeat three times

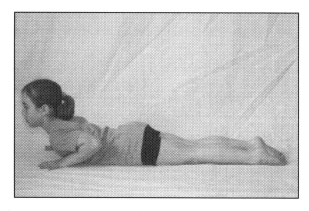 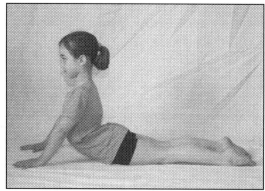

Compass – La boussole

- Stand, feet together
- Inhale, raise both hands overhead, intertwine fingers, pointing upward with index fingers
- Exhale, bend forward (north), inhale coming up
- Exhale, bend backward (south), inhale coming up
- Exhale, bend to the left (west), inhale coming up
- Exhale, bend to the right (east), inhale coming up
- Repeat series one more time

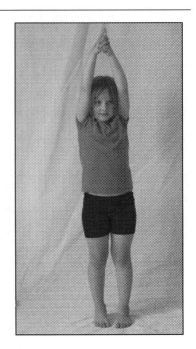

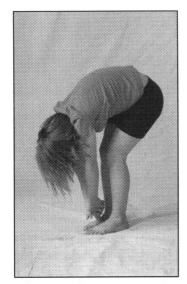

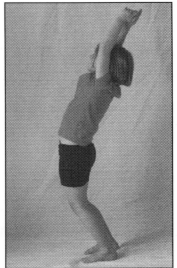

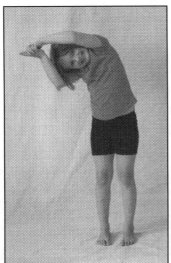

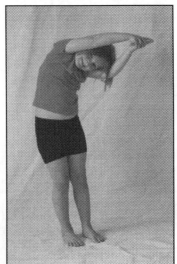

Corpse – Le cadavre

(Savasana)

- Lie down on your back
- Place your hands by your hips, palms facing upward
- Spread your feet a bit wider than hip-distance apart
- Close your eyes, relax and breathe deeply and evenly

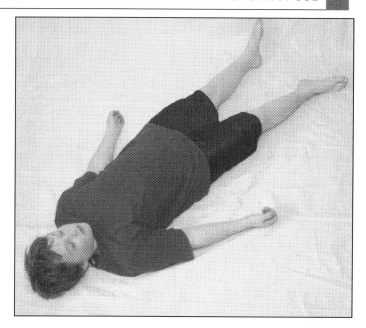

Cow-Faced – Le visage de la vache

(Gomukhasana)

- Sit, bring the left foot back to the right hip
- Lift the right foot over the left knee trying to align the knees
- Reach your right arm down and behind with the hand coming up to the middle back
- Reach your left arm high over head then bend the elbow hoping to touch the right fingers behind the back
- Repeat on the other side

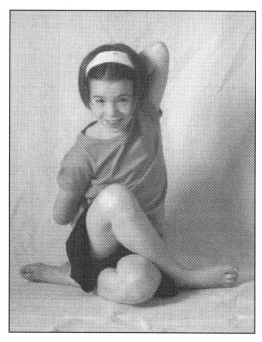

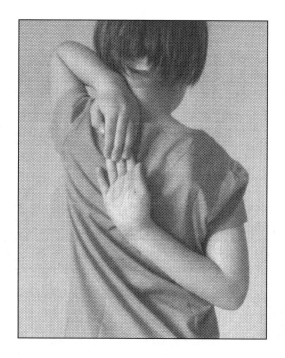

Crocodile – Le crocodile

(Chataranga)

- Kneel on all fours in **Table** position
- Straighten your legs behind you in **Plank** position
- Slowly lower your body, keeping your elbows in touching your ribs; hold off of the floor for an active, hunting crocodile
- Relax on the floor for a crocodile basking in the sun

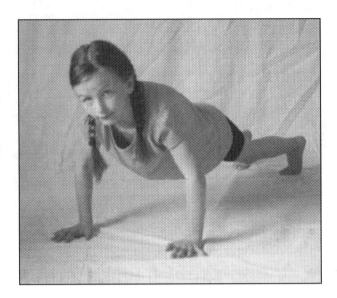

Crow – Le corbeau

(Bakasana)

- Squat with knees wide apart
- Place both hands on the floor, fingers spread
- Try to get your knees up as high as possible on your upper arm
- Slowly put your weight on your arms
- Lift one foot, then the other, then try to lift both feet, balancing on your hands
- This is one of the most difficult poses included in this book, but there is almost always one student who can do it
- Emphasize the worth of trying and practising hard

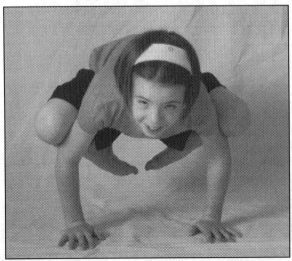 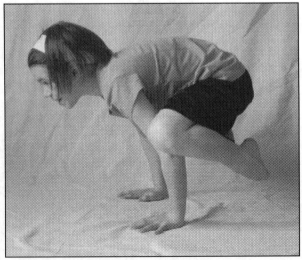

Dancer – Le roi de la danse

(Natarajasana)

- Stand, feet hip-distance apart
- Bending the right knee, grasp the inside of the right foot with the right hand
- Raise the left hand overhead
- Lift the right foot behind and up, allow the torso to move forward, opening the chest, balancing on one foot
- Repeat on the opposite side

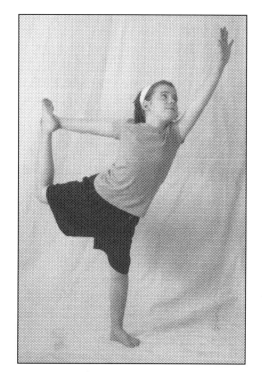

Deer – Le cerf

(Marichiyasana II)

- Sit, feet stretched out of the floor in front of you
- Bend the right leg placing the foot a hand's span from the left thigh
- Hug your knee with both arms and sit tall
- Place the right hand on the floor behind you, inhale as you reach up with the left hand
- Exhale and twist your torso to hug your right knee with the left arm, look behind you
- Release, returning to center
- Repeat on the other side

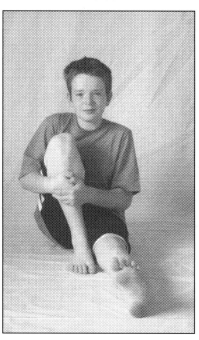 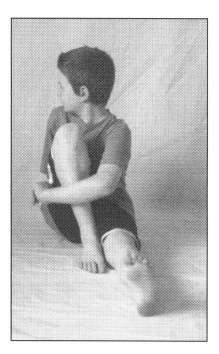

Dolphin – Le dauphin

- Kneel tall, intertwine your fingers, bend your elbows
- Place your forearms on the floor in front of you, elbows below your shoulders in a variation of **Table** position, arms making a triangle on the floor
- Curl your toes under
- Lift your hips high, let your head hang down, not touching the floor
- To make your Dolphin swim, lower your hips and bring your head up into a variation of **Plank** position, then lift and lower, lift and lower as your Dolphin frolics in the waves
- Come down and relax

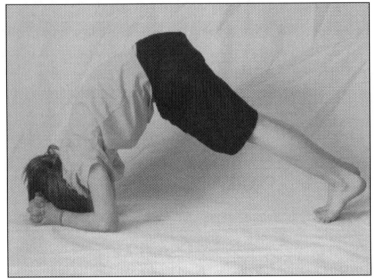

Donkey Kicks – Coup de sabots de l'âne

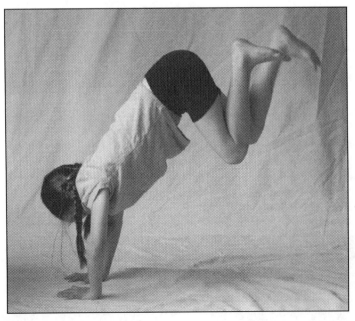

- Kneel on all fours in **Table** position
- Kick your legs up behind you as high as you can
- Repeat several times, braying like a donkey

Downward Dog – Le chien à la baisse

(Adho mukha svanasana)

- Kneel on all fours in **Table** position
- Curl your toes under
- Lift your hips high and back, extend your arms, keeping your palms flat on the floor
- Let your head hang down, look at your navel
- Wag your tail, lift one leg, then lift the other leg, bark like a dog
- Come down and relax

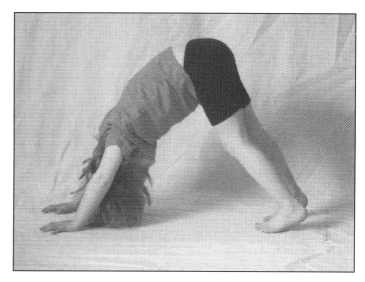

Eagle – L'aigle

(Garudasana)

- Stand, feet together
- Find a spot on the floor to focus on
- Bending the left leg, cross the right leg overtop
- Lift the left arm in front of you, elbow bent, fingers reaching up
- Circle the right arm under the left arm, trying to bring your hands to meet
- Hold and breathe, sinking the hips, lifting the arms
- Count down (3, 2, 1) and fly away, releasing the pose, spreading the arms wide
- Repeat on the other side

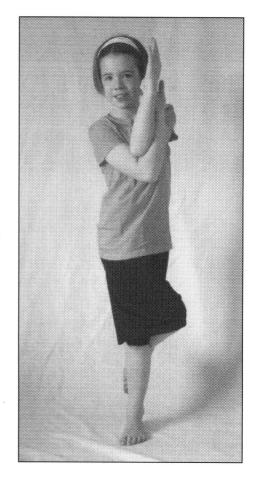

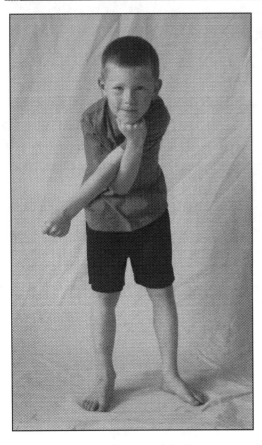

Elephant – L'éléphant

- Imitate an elephant
- Possibilities include making a trunk with your arms by holding your chin with one hand and putting the other hand through the opening; using your trunk to pick up balls off the floor and trying to bring them to your mouth; using your trunk to scratch your back (remember both sides); greeting other elephants by shaking trunks; trumpeting like an elephant

Fish – Le poisson
(Matsyasana)

- Lie down on your back, hands by your hips or underneath your buttocks
- Gently roll onto the top of your head, opening the chest, keeping the hips on the floor
- Make fish lips and enjoy looking at the world upside down
- As you release, be sure not to lift the head, but gently roll back to lying flat

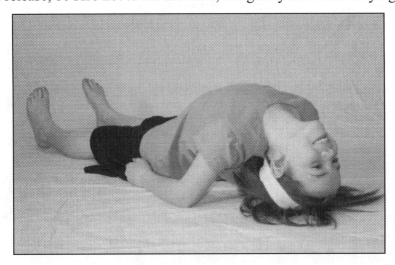

Gate – Le portail

(Parighasana)

- Kneel tall, extend the right leg out straight to the side, toes forward
- Keep your shoulders and hips squared to the front
- Place the right hand on the right leg
- Reach overhead with the left arm, keep reaching over toward the right, feeling a lovely stretch along the left side
- Repeat on the other side

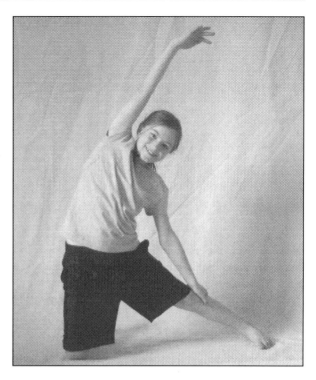

Growing Flower – La fleur croissante

- Crouch down on the floor, making yourself as small as possible just like a seed
- Imagine the rain falling on you, the sun warming you
- Begin to slowly grow, unfolding your body, stretching up to the sky, and blooming with a beautiful smile

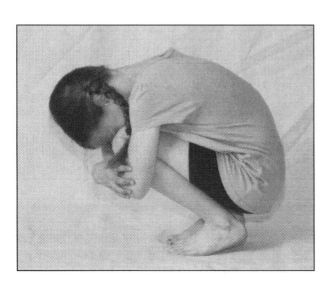

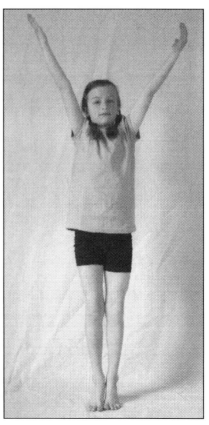

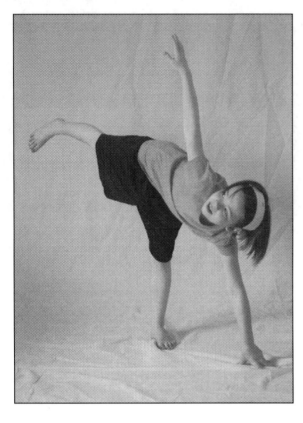

Half Moon – La demi-lune
(Ardha chandrasana)

- Stand, left foot in front of the right foot
- Bend your knees and place your fingertips on the floor in front of you
- Lift your right leg straight behind you, aiming for 90 degrees from the ground
- Raise the right arm, stretching for the sky, twisting your torso
- Tuck the left or lower shoulder under, stacking the shoulders one atop the other
- Breathe and try to look up without falling over
- Repeat on the other side

Happy Baby – Le bébé très heureux
(Ananda Balasana)

- Sit, grasping the inside of your feet with your hands
- Roll onto your back, feet to the sky
- Coo, giggle, and make happy baby noises, then roll back to sitting

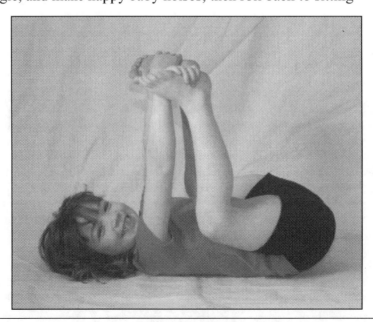

Hero – Le héros

(Virasana)

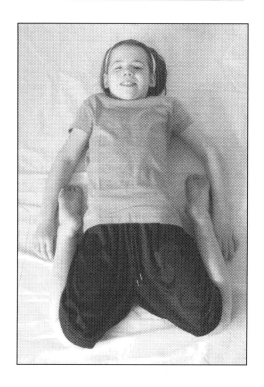

- Kneel low; if this is comfortable move onto the next step
- Slide your feet to the side and sit between your feet, be sure toes are pointing back, not out to the side; if this is comfortable move onto the next step
- Lie down on your back, hands either by your sides or overhead
- Relax and breathe deeply

Inchworm – L'arpentuese

- Have the group stand along one wall
- Bend over so that your hands are flat on the floor, knees will be bent slightly
- Walk hands as far forward as possible into **Plank** position
- Walk feet up to meet hands
- Repeat with hands and legs, taking turns walking until students cross the room
- Return to your mat

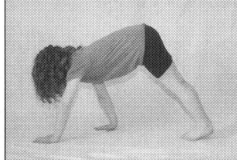

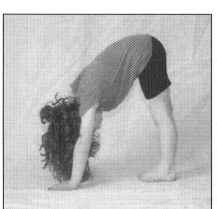

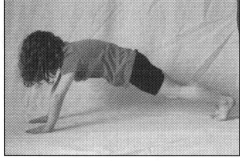

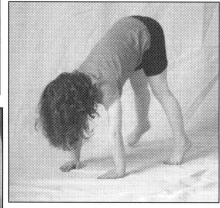

King Cobra – Le cobra royal

(Bhujangasana)

- Begin by performing **Cobra** pose
- Try to get your feet to touch your head—this is challenging, but there always seems to be one or two individuals who can accomplish it thanks to natural flexibility—celebrate this!

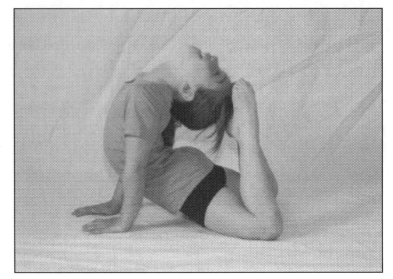

Lion – Le lion

(Simhasana)

- Sit cross-legged or kneel low
- Think of something negative in your life, squeeze it in, clasping the hands, crunching up the face, tight, tight
- Let it go by extending the arms forward and roaring loudly, sticking the tongue out
- Repeat three times

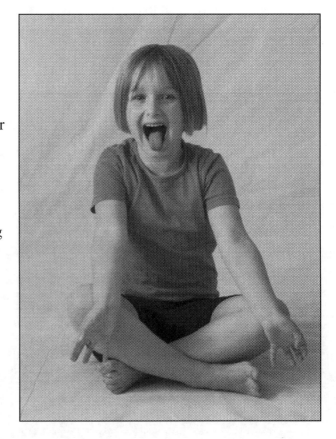

Locust – La locuste
(Salabhasana)

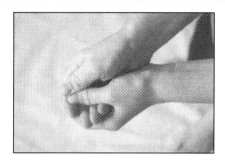

- Demonstrate how to bump the ball for volleyball, one hand on top of the other, thumbs folded in and touching
- Lie on your back beside your mat, put your hands into the bump position
- Roll onto your stomach and shoulders, hands down by your groin; the legs will rise higher when your weight is more on your shoulders
- Lift the right leg, lift the left leg, lift both legs

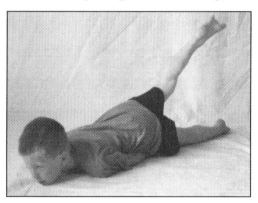
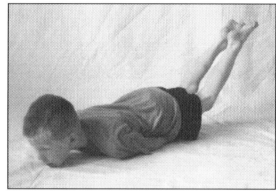

Lotus – Le lotus
(Padmasana)

- Sit cross-legged; if this is comfortable, move onto the next step
- Gently lift one foot and bring it close to the opposite hip (**Half Lotus**); if this is comfortable, move onto the next step
- Lift the other foot and bring it close to the opposite hip (**Full Lotus**)

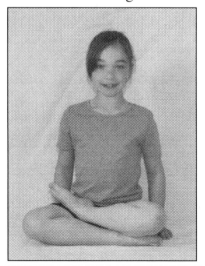
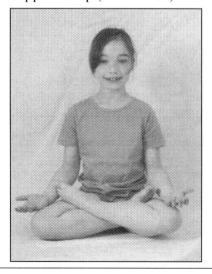

Monkey – Le singe

- Imitate a monkey—by yourself or with a partner as a mirror
- Possibilities include jumping like a chimp; bending so that knuckles can be used for walking; scratching armpits; shaking arms; chattering teeth; pursing lips; picking flees (grooming); chest-beating; saying 'oo-oo, ah-ah'

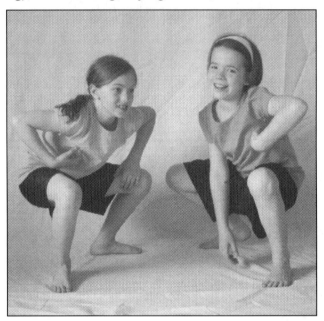

Moon Buggy – Le véhicule lunaire

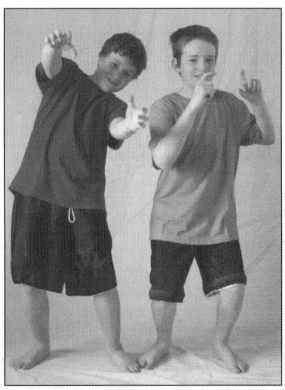

- With a partner, climb into a "moon buggy"
- Decide what activities and experiments you will do as you drive around the moon—driving, taking pictures, gathering samples
- Remember the moon's surface is bumpy and filled with craters large and small
- Return to your mat

Moon Walk – Promenade sur la lune

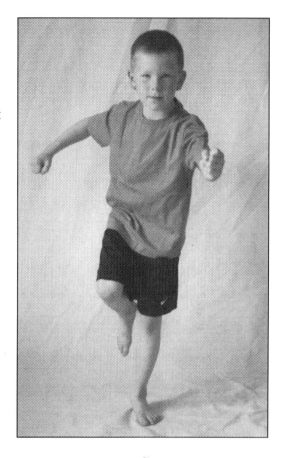

- Imagine you weigh 1/6 your current weight (approximately 50 lbs = 8 lbs, 75 lbs = 12.5 lbs, 100 lbs = 16 lbs)
- Walk around the room with little gravitational force, bounding lightly, feet making no sound, floating through the air
- Return to your mat

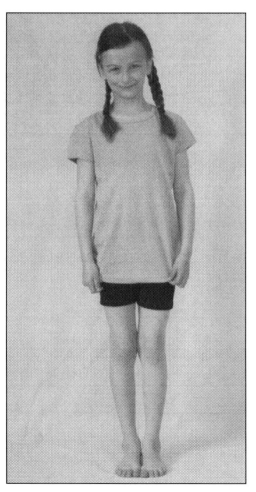

Mountain – La montagne
(Tadasana)

- Stand, feet together or hip-width apart, evenly balanced on the three points of the foot: big toe knuckle, little toe knuckle, centre of the heel
- Engage your quadriceps (thigh muscles) by pulling up on the knees
- Roll your shoulders up, then back and down
- Keep your hands by your sides, palms facing in
- Imagine someone zipping you up from your knees to the crown of your head
- Stand tall and immovable like a mountain

Phone – Le téléphone

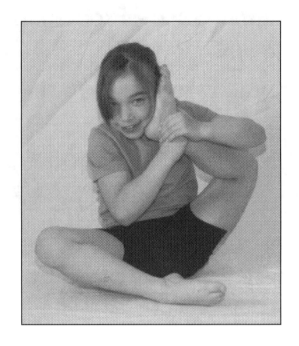

- Sit cross-legged
- Grab your right foot and bring it to your right ear
- Chat, then release
- Repeat on the other side

Pigeon – Le pigeon
(Eka pada rajakapotasana)

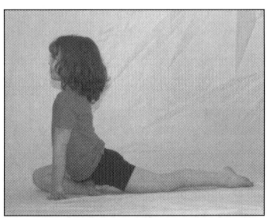

- Sit cross-legged, extend your right leg straight behind you
- Square your shoulders and hips to the front
- Lie down overtop the bent left leg, resting your head in your hands
- Relax and coo like a pigeon
- Straighten back up; if this is comfortable, move onto the next step
- Reaching back with your right hand, clasp the right foot by bending the knee
- Breathe, open the chest and hips, release
- Repeat on the other side

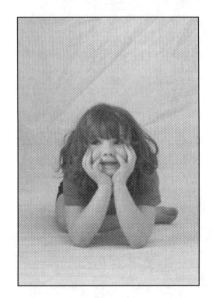

Plough – La charrue
(Halasana)

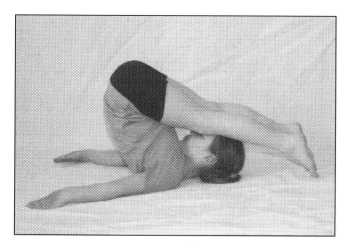

- Lie on your back
- Roll your feet over your head, extending the legs until they touch the floor or a chair
- The weight should be on the shoulders, not the neck
- Support the back with the hands and breathe
- Gently return to lying flat on your back

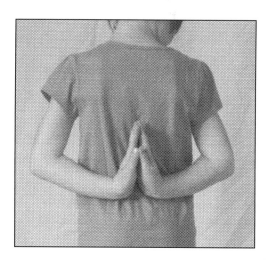

Pyramid – La pyramide
(Parsvottanasana)

- Stand with your right foot in front of the left, feet hip distance apart
- Place your hands in **Reverse Prayer** position with palms touching behind your back, fingers pointed up, or simply hold your elbows behind your back
- Inhale and lengthen the body, exhale bending forward over the right leg, aiming your chin for the shin, keep both legs straight
- Breathe, on an inhale return to standing
- Switch the feet and repeat

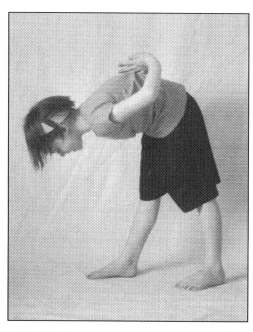

Rabbit – Le lapin

(Sasangasana)

- Kneel tall, intertwine your fingers, bend your elbows
- Place your forearms on the floor in front of you, elbows below your shoulders in a variation of **Table** position, arms making a triangle on the floor
- Place the crown of your head in the hole in the centre of the triangle made by your arms
- Curl your toes under
- Lift your hips high, pushing into the floor with your arms so your neck doesn't collapse
- If it's comfortable, walk your feet slightly toward your head
- Come down and relax

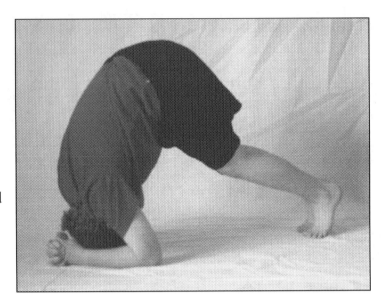

Ragdoll – La poupée de chiffon

- Stand, feet slightly apart
- Flop over, head and arms hanging down, bend your knees if you want
- Relax and breathe
- Slowly return to standing by rolling up

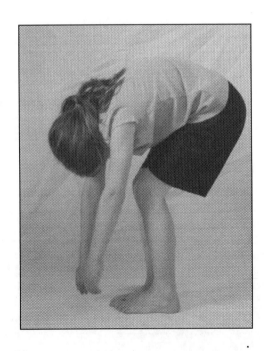

Robot – Le robot

- Imitate a robot: walking, talking, moving arms, legs, and head

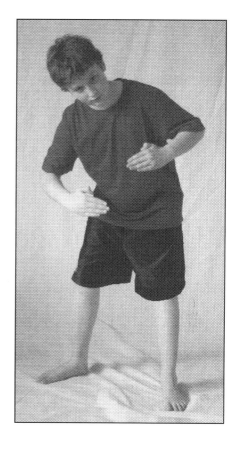

Rock the Baby – Bercer l'enfant

- Sit cross-legged
- Place your right foot in the crook of the left elbow
- Wrap your right arm around the right knee, intertwining fingers
- Rock your 'baby' forward and back, side to side, release
- Repeat on the other side

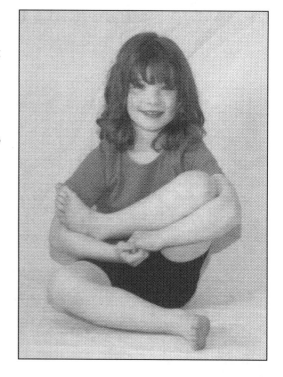

Rocket – La fusée

- Stand, feet slightly apart
- Inhale, raise both hands overhead, intertwine fingers, pointing upward with index fingers
- Bend knees into a deep squat
- Countdown 10, 9, 8, 7, 6, 5, 4, 3, 2, 1, Blastoff!
- Jump high, reaching for the stars

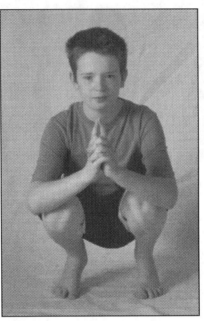
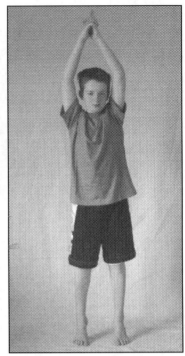

Shower – Étirements de la douche

- Stand and imagine warm water pouring down on your head
- Alternatively use your fingers to imitate drops of water falling on your body, tapping your fingers on your head and working your way down over your neck, shoulders, arms, chest, belly, and legs
- Pretend to wash your body with exaggerated movements: belly, back, arms, legs, toes
- Turn the 'water' off and pretend to dry yourself off with a towel

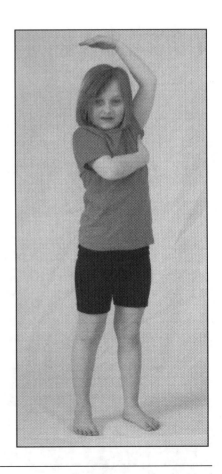

Sphinx – Le sphinx

- Lie on your stomach
- Place your hands in a **Sphinx** position, elbows below the shoulders, forearms extended forward
- Pull the shoulders down, creating space between the shoulders and ears
- Think Sphinx-like thoughts while you enjoy a simple backbend

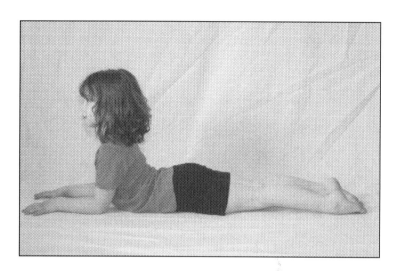

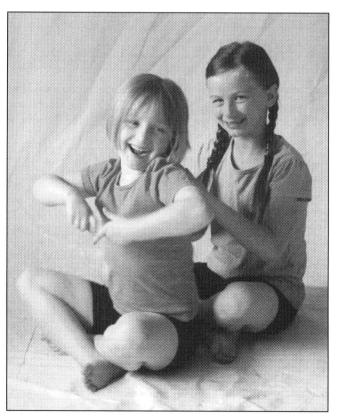

Spider – L'araignée

- In partners, one person be the 'child,' the other be the 'spider'
- Sit with the spider behind the child
- Sing 'Eensy, Weensy Spider' as the spider crawls their fingers up and down the child's back and the child does the actions to the song
- Switch roles and repeat

Star (body) – L'étoile (le corps)

- Lie on your back
- Stretch the right hand overhead on the floor
- Stretch the left hand out at shoulder height along the floor
- Lift the left leg straight up
- Cross the left leg over to the right, creating a twist in the spine
- Stretch strongly into all points of your star
- Relax and return to lying flat on your back
- Repeat on the other side

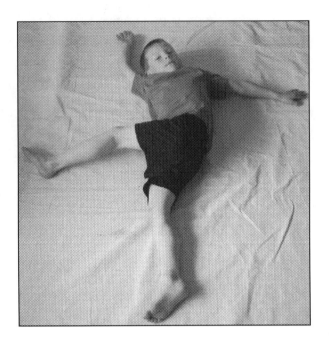

Star (hand) – L'étoile (la main)

- Hold one hand out and imagine there is a star in your palm
- Slowly make your star shine, bright, bright, brighter
- Back off a little (70% intensity is a safe zone)
- Discuss personal energy and working within safe boundaries
- Discuss having a star within that shines brightly, that we share our light with others, that others follow our light

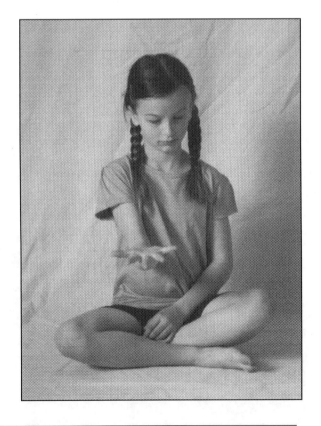

Tent – La tente

(Prasarita Padottanasana)

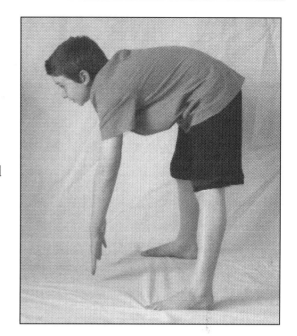

- Stand, legs wide apart, both feet flat on the floor, toes pointed slightly in to protect the lower back
- Place your hands on your hips, inhale and extend your body
- Exhale and bend forward, allowing the hands to touch the ground in front of you
- Inhale and extend the body, exhale and increase the forward bend, keeping the legs straight
- After a few breaths, slowly return to standing on an inhale

Tiptoe – La pointe des pieds

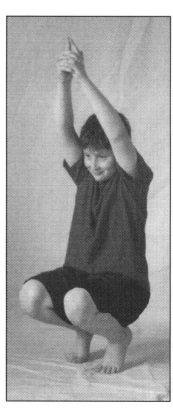

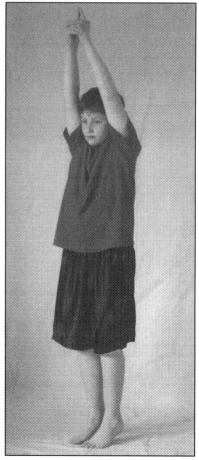

- Stand, feet slightly apart
- Raise your hands overhead, intertwine your fingers, index fingers pointing up
- Lift onto your tiptoes
- While staying on your tiptoes, lower yourself to a squat, keeping your balance
- Still on tiptoes, raise your body
- Return to standing, feet flat

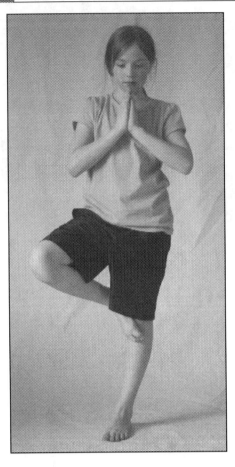

Tree – L'arbre
(Vriksasana)

- Stand, feet together; find something on the floor two feet in front of you to focus on
- Extend your arms at shoulder height out to the side
- Lift the right foot, turning the knee out; place the right foot above or below the knee
- Imagine your toes are the roots, your standing leg is the trunk, your arms and bent leg are branches
- To test your balance:
  1. Bring your arms to **Prayer** position in front of your heart
  2. Raise your arms overhead
  3. Look up to your hands

Turtle – La tortue
(Kurmasana)

- Sit, legs bent but wide apart
- Work your torso between your knees, wrapping your arms under your legs and grasping your ankles
- Try to straighten your legs and lower your torso to the ground, hiding within your turtle shell

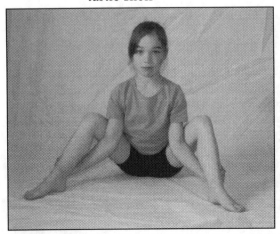

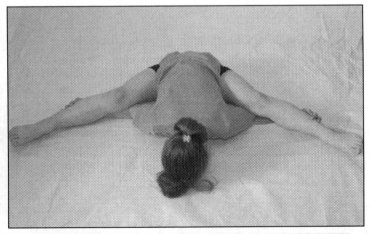

Two Scoops – Deux boules de crème glacée

- In pairs, have one partner perform **Child's** pose, being certain to lower their hips and make their back as flat as possible
- The other partner performs **Child's** pose on top of their partner, making two scoops of ice cream with their bodies
- Switch roles and repeat

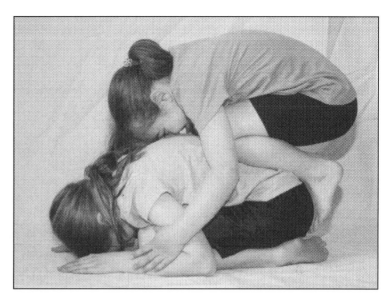

Warrior – Le guerrier
(Virabhadrasana II)

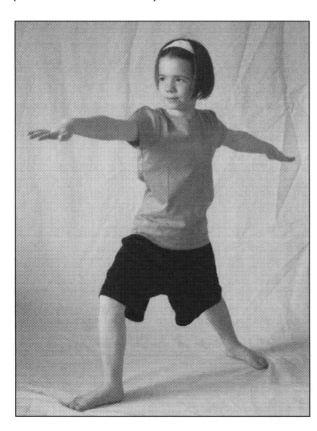

- Stand, legs wide apart
- Keep your hips and shoulders in line with your feet, don't allow the back hip to roll forward
- Turn your left foot in slightly; this is your brake
- Turn your right foot out 90 degrees; this is your forward foot
- Inhale and raise your arms out to the sides at shoulder height, with arms actively stretching
- Exhale and gently bend your forward knee, watching the ankle for a 90-degree angle
- Gaze at your forward hand and think 'warrior' thoughts: I am brave, I am strong
- Return to standing
- Repeat on the other side by first switching the feet (right becomes the brake, left becomes the forward foot), then follow directions

Washing Machine – La machine à laver

- Sit cross-legged
- Cross your arms over your chest, hands at opposite shoulders
- Twist left and right like a washing machine agitator as you huff out "swish, swish, swish" from side to side
- Follow this up with **Dryer** pose by rolling your arms in front of you, fast for dry and slow for fluff

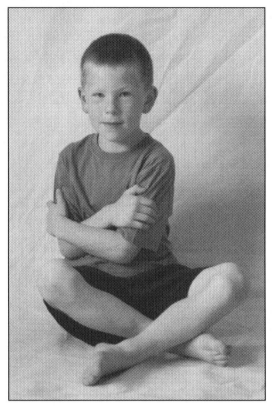

Wheel – La roue

(Urdva dhanurasana)

- Lie on your back, legs bent with feet close to hips
- Circle your arms so fingers are tucked under shoulders, thumbs close to ears
- Push up into a back bend and breathe
- Come down gently and rest

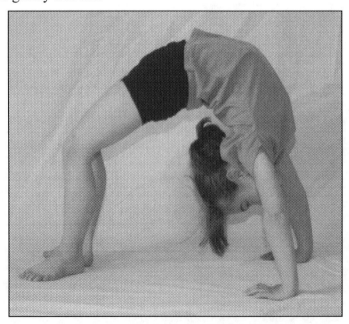

Chapter 5   Breathing

When the breath wanders, the mind also is unsteady. But when the breath is calmed, the mind too will be still, and the yogi achieves long life. Therefore, one should learn to control the breath. — Hatha Yoga Pradipika

Understanding the Breath

The respiratory system is unique in that it is both involuntary (something that occurs without conscious thought) and voluntary (something that we can control by lengthening, shortening, or holding the breath). In yoga, the control of the breath is known as *pranayama.*

Our breath is synonymous with our life. Life enters with first inhalation and leaves with final exhalation. The breath serves as an extension of *prana*, or life force, as it moves in the body. This gentle rhythm is our constant companion.

When we are born our breath is full, flowing and uninhibited. It is a whole body experience. This happens as the pelvic floor expands and descends on inhalations, and contracts and lifts on exhalations. The collarbone lifts and rolls upward on inhalation and descends on exhalation. The upper arms externally rotate on inhalation and internally rotate on exhalation.

Most people do not fully utilize their breath, compromising their physical and emotional health. The first step to remedy this is breath awareness: simply observing the breath. Is it erratic, short, long, or shallow? Can you maintain focus on the breath or are you easily distracted? See the exercise **Observing the Breath** (p.104) for specifics on how to accomplish this.

The breath rejuvenates the body, allowing oxygen into the blood stream to bathe each cell with its life-giving force. Internal organs, all the body systems, the brain, etc., require oxygen to perform their proper function.

By learning to control our breathing, we can influence our emotional state, our ability to concentrate, and the way energy moves in our bodies. Breathing exercises develop the ability to calm and control the breath, allowing us to focus the mind and manage emotions.

Pranayama practice strengthens all of the muscles involved in breathing, increases respiratory efficiency, and helps to expand the capacity of the lungs.

Most of us breathe very shallowly into the lungs and don't give much thought to how we breathe. Yoga breathing exercises focus the attention on the breath and teach us how to better use our lungs, which benefits the entire body. Certain types of breathing exercises can also help clear the nasal passages and even calm the central nervous system, which has both physical and mental benefits.

Yoga for Asthma

Children with asthma are encouraged to participate in physical activities. In fact, physical activity will help prevent asthmatics from becoming isolated, withdrawn, and physically unconditioned. In particular, movement education, such as yoga, is beneficial for students with asthma because it provides an anaerobic activity with warm-up and cool-down periods.

Yoga exercises, including *asanas*, breathing exercises, and relaxation techniques put you in control of your mind and emotions. This increases relaxation and allows you to breathe easier. This will also help your lungs work better and enhance airflow during asthma episodes.

Yogic practices result in more anxiety reduction than do drugs. Yoga gives an asthmatic access to their own internal experience and helps them pinpoint possible causes of their ailment, i.e., find their own triggers. This comes through increased self-awareness. Simple yogic practices help regulate breathing patterns, as well as enhance lung functioning. The result is that many asthmatics are able to better manage their condition by allaying their fears and anxieties.

Yoga also has a stabilizing effect on the body's immune system. It is now proven that the regular and consistent practice of yoga raises the body's tolerance to infection as well as its local resistance to infections in the respiratory tract. Yogic rest and relaxation reduce the nervous system's overall activity, leading to remarkable recovery.

Breathing is an integral part of yoga and tremendous importance is placed on proper and effective breathing techniques. These yogic techniques help to strengthen the lungs and ensure that we breathe fully and properly. Yoga techniques can ensure that we utilize almost one hundred per cent of our lung capacity and help to preclude the possibility of respiratory ailments, including asthma.

Yoga also helps to calm the mind and bring it in sync with the body. It promotes relaxation and helps to alleviate stress and tension. It can help one to understand the emotional and physical triggers that induce an asthma attack, and thereby avoid them. Truly, yoga can be a tremendous aid to asthmatics.

Please continue to take any prescribed medication and be sure that your school has a personal Asthma Action Plan in place. The Canadian Lung Association (visit www.lung.ca) and the web site www.asthmainschools.com are terrific places to look for more information and resources in helping students with asthma. Specific exercises and breathing techniques for asthma relief can be found at www.yogainmyschool.com.

Basics to Remember

- **Breathe in and out through the nose**
- **An inhalation is breathing in, an exhalation is breathing out**
- **Generally, you expand on an inhalation and contract on an exhalation**
- **Breathe slowly, deeply, and with thought**

Breathing Exercises

Air Walk

Lie down on your back. Begin to walk in the air. Keep your right leg straight and lift it up as you lift the left arm. Breathe in as you lift, breathe out as your arm and leg go down. Then inhale again and lift the left leg and the right arm together. Exhale down. Keep going. Stretch straight up toward the sky. If this is hard, remember: you tell your brain what you want it to do! Air Walk balances the two sides of your brain, and helps you think better.

Counting the Breath

Lie in **Corpse** pose. Allow your breath to settle, listening carefully. Observe the inhalation and exhalation, counting each to determine its length. Make them equal in length. If you inhale to a count of four, exhale to a count of four. Start to extend each breath. Try to count to six or eight, keeping the breath even and unforced.

Extending the Breath

Lie in **Corpse** pose. Let your breath settle, listening carefully. Count how long each inhalation and exhalation takes. Start to make your exhalations longer, until they are twice as long as the inhalations. Repeat several times. Now focus on the pause between each breath. Gently hold your breath at the top of each inhalation, exhale. Aim to eventually hold your breath three times longer than the inhalation. Use the 1:3:2 ratio where you inhale to a count of four, hold for 12, and exhale for eight. Pause gently, continue with natural breathing.

Observing the Breath

Lie in **Corpse** pose or sit cross-legged with your back straight. Close your eyes and place your hands on your chest and abdomen to help you feel the movement of the breath. Listen to the flow of air into and out of your body. Visualize a particle of air flowing into your nostrils, going down your throat, into your lungs and entering the bloodstream. As you exhale, reverse this pathway. How does your breath feel? Is it rough, smooth, fast, slow, even, or uneven? Do not control the breath, simply observe. If your mind wanders, bring your focus back gently to the movement of each breath.

Swimming Stuffies

Lie in **Corpse** pose with a small stuffed animal on your abdomen. Close your eyes. Inhale and exhale, allowing the breath to originate deep in the belly. Feel the inhalation expand the abdomen, lifting the stuffed animal. On the exhale, the abdomen condenses and the stuffy dips. Make your stuffed animal swim on this wave of breath for several rounds.

Take Five

Sit comfortably. Lift one finger at a time as you breathe in through your nose and count in your mind: 1, 2, 3, 4, 5. Pause for a second. As you exhale, count backward (5, 4, 3, 2, 1), putting down a finger for each number. Repeat two or three times.

Three-Stage Breathing or Diaphragmatic Breathing

Lie in **Corpse** pose. Relax and allow your body to sink into the ground. Become aware of your breathing. Begin deep in the belly. Inhale expanding the abdomen, exhale pushing the air out of the abdomen. Continue for a few rounds. Next, expand the belly, then the ribs, allowing them to pull outward like a balloon inflating. Exhale from the belly, followed by the ribs. Again begin in the abdomen, then expand the ribs, breathing into the back ribs this time. Exhale belly first, then ribs. Finally add in the upper chest. Start deep in the belly, then expand the ribs, next fill the lungs all the way up to the clavicles or collar bones. Exhale starting in the belly, relax the ribs, and squeeze all the air out of the upper chest. Repeat. Return to a normal breath, not making any extra effort or attention.

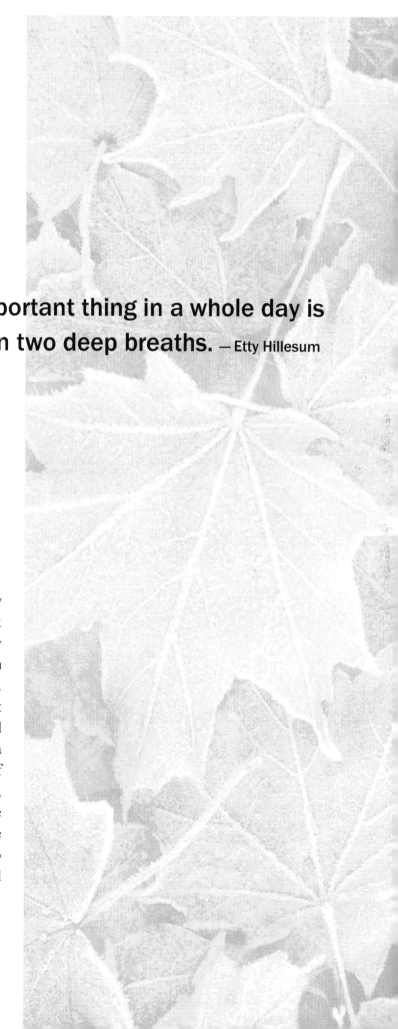

Chapter 6   Relaxation

Sometimes the most important thing in a whole day is the rest we take between two deep breaths. — Etty Hillesum

The Need to Relax

Most people are so busy in today's society they simply don't have the time to relax properly. Furthermore, they don't know how to go about doing it. We all know relaxation is essential for our health and well-being. The constant stresses of daily living affect the body physically, emotionally, and behaviourally. These can manifest in a variety of ways and can lead to all kinds of problems, such as depression, headaches, under- or overeating, insomnia, and extreme emotions such as anger or frustration. The good news, however, is that you can undo stress, since it is primarily a self-generated pressure based on feelings and perceptions.

Relaxation counters the effects of stress by allowing the immune system to recover and function more effectively. This includes restoring organs and glands, reducing muscle tension and encouraging deeper, more rhythmic breathing. It helps lower blood pressure, and so decreases the likelihood of stroke and heart attack.

In addition, it provides an emotional break from stressors, and lowers the activity in the limbic system (or emotional centre) of the brain. Relaxation is accompanied by a pleasurable, good feeling. It renews depleted energy supplies and restores normal functioning levels in general. Each time you relax, right-hemispheric brain activity is increased, which results in a clearer, calmer state of mind.

Children, in particular, are in desperate need of learning to relax. They are over-stimulated, over-scheduled, and are not provided with the tools, or allowed the time, to be quiet and become acquainted with themselves.

Teachers are in a unique position to teach relaxation techniques and immediately apply them to their students' advantage. Incorporating relaxation techniques is easily done in five- to ten-minute segments, and can greatly benefit all within the classroom. Ideally, relaxation is conducted daily at a routine time, but any efforts in this direction will produce results.

Simple relaxation techniques will contribute to improved verbal and spatial memory, reduced anxiety, enhanced creativity, and increased clarity. They will aid in self-awareness development, encourage positive

coping strategies, clear the mind for full concentration at a given task, and decrease impulsiveness and aggression. This definitely describes a classroom where all are emotionally, physically, and mentally prepared to get to the serious and fulfilling work at hand.

> **Don't underestimate the value of doing nothing, of just going along, listening to all the things you can't hear, and not bothering.**
> — Pooh's Little Instruction Book, inspired by A.A. Milne

Affirmations

Affirmations are short phrases that affect the subconscious mind and mould feelings, behaviours, and attitudes. They help to reprogram existing behaviours and thoughts, leading one to greater success and positive action.

Most of us have an internal dialogue that is often primarily negative. We repeat negative statements in our minds without even being aware of what we are doing or thinking. Telling ourselves that we are lazy, often make mistakes, can't do something, or will fail, brings those exact undesirable results into being. This negative self-talk sets us up for failure, drains our energy, and exaggerates real and perceived weaknesses and shortcomings. The use of positive affirmations is a technique to change this negativity into something positive and empowering. It is a process of becoming aware of daily thoughts and choosing to think positive, self-affirming ones

Children generally have no idea in regards to their internal dialogue. Teaching them to pay attention to their thoughts and to focus their efforts on positive attitudes and desires provides a powerful life skill.

The words in an affirmation help to focus on the aim, objective, or situation one wants to achieve or create. They have three elements:

- They are phrased in the first person present. For example, "I am calm and relaxed."
- They are positive. For example, "My body is healthy and functioning in a good way."
- They are specific. For example, "I contribute to class by sharing my ideas."

By affirming what you want in life, you mentally and emotionally make it true. By repeating the words you focus your mind on your goal, and create a mental image of the desired result. These mental images imprint on the subconscious mind and transform habits, behaviour, reactions, and attitude.

Affirmations are very influential and can have enormous impact on personal success. Affirmations can be used with poses to reinforce their benefits. An affirmation for **Wheel** pose may be, "I am flexible. My heart is open. My brain is alert." Repeating affirmations numerous times while in a relaxed state, such as **Corpse** pose, has tremendous power and influence.

Repeating affirmations often, and writing them down on small cards or post-it notes which are placed in highly visible locations, such as the bathroom mirror or school desk, are two additional ways to access the benefits of these powerful, transformative phrases.

Seated Relaxation

Sit comfortably in a chair. You may lean forward with your head on the desk/table or sit tall, whichever is more comfortable. Alternatively (if space allows), lay on the floor on your back, feet hip-width apart, palms facing up, chin relaxed. Close your eyes. Take a few deep breaths, allowing the breath to lengthen and deepen with each exhalation. Feel as if you are sinking: your limbs becoming heavier. Allow the tension to leave your body. Without rushing, work through one of the guided relaxation exercises which follow. When finished, rest, eyes closed, for a moment. Slowly, mentally come back to your surroundings, wiggle your fingers, wiggle your toes, open your eyes, and sit up. Enjoy the rest of your day with renewed vigour and mental acuity.

Guided Imagery Relaxation Exercises

The following visualization exercises are effective at reducing the negative effects of stress, of inducing the relaxation response, and helping individuals cope with life's challenges. They are similar to inducing a vivid day dream and help individuals to access their inner wisdom. Practise them during a **Seated Relaxation** or **Corpse** pose (*savasana*) after a yoga session.

Bathing Beauty

Bring a deep, hot, jacuzzi bath to mind. Add in some scented bath beads or bubbles if you so desire. Imagine a few candles lit around the tub, the lights are dim. Slowly slip your feet into the water, then your legs, your torso. Stop there for a moment and breathe. Now, lie back, sink all the way up to your neck. Rest your head on the back of the tub. Let your arms and legs float, resting and relaxing, enjoying the warmth and comfort.

Beach Bunny

Imagine that you are sunbathing on a warm, sandy beach. See the palm trees swaying in the gentle breeze. Smell the salt air. Hear the waves as they lap at the shore and listen as the seabirds call to one another. Feel the sun soak into your skin, warming and relaxing every part of your body: your legs, your arms, your torso, your throat and face. Relax and enjoy the feeling of being on the beach with no one making any demands on your time or energy.

Beautiful Garden

Visualize a garden filled with plants and flowers—splashes of green are interspersed with yellow, orange, red, pink, and white. Wisps of clouds float in a blue sky. Golden sunlight filters down through the trees. You enjoy its warmth on your face and hands. Smell the roses and honeysuckle. Hear the buzz of insects and birds chirping and singing. Feel the wind as it rustles the leaves. Tune into the scents and sounds, enjoying the bounty of the garden.

Bird Feeder

Remember lying on the grass under the trees on a lovely summer day. Relax as you watch the wind ruffle the leaves. Feel the gentle sway of the branches. There are birds flying around, hopping from branch to branch. In your upturned hands, there is a bit of bird seed. As you lie perfectly still, the birds gain courage. Keep breathing slowly and smoothly and they will come and eat from your hands.

Consult an Animal Guide

Imagine a kind, loving, protective animal. It may be a bear, dog, horse, eagle, or other animal that you love and admire. This animal possesses great wisdom. Follow your animal guide as it leads you to solutions to problems. Maybe your animal helps you be brave, or patient, or helps you to fall asleep. Allow your animal into your life whenever you are upset or stressed. It will help you to face your challenges with courage and love.

Favourite Colour

What is your favourite colour? Bring it to mind. Think of various things that are your favourite colour: a flower, the sky, the mountains, your favourite food, a gemstone, the eyes of a loved one. As you inhale, imagine a wave of beautiful, vibrant colour streaming into your body, filling every space. As you exhale, imagine all the dull dirty grey inside you is flowing out. Continue to fill your body, deeply and profoundly as you breathe in, while eliminating all the negativity as you breathe out. After a few rounds, enjoy the sensation of energy that fills you, and keep this with you throughout your day.

Floating on a Cloud

Imagine that a fluffy white cloud floats out of the sky, down toward you. It rests beside you. Your body floats up and onto the cloud. It's as soft as the softest bed, cushioning your body. The cloud slowly lifts off the ground and rises into the sky. It floats for a while and you can enjoy the view, the weightlessness, and the peace. Slowly the cloud comes back down, returning you safely to the earth. Your body remembers that feeling of floating weightlessly throughout the day.

Goals

Think about the achievements you would like to accomplish in one month, one year, five years, and even ten years from now. Let your ideas flow naturally. Think of various categories: family and relationships, career, health, and personal development. Think of steps you can take to fulfill these goals. Be realistic but allow yourself to stretch to your full potential.

Hot-Air-Balloon

In your mind's eye, visualize a brightly coloured hot-air balloon anchored to the ground. The balloon seems inviting—a great way to escape the pressures of the day. Climb into the wicker basket. You look down, trying to figure out how to take off, and realize the basket is weighed down by stones—these stones represent various problems in your life. You heave the stones over the side, one by one. The basket soon starts to wobble and then drift upward. High up in the sky you feel free. Spend a few moments drifting along with the breeze before returning to earth.

In and Out

Concentrate on your breath. As you inhale, imagine that all the good things you want,

like happiness and peace, are flowing into your body along with the breath. As you exhale, imagine all the bad things, like tension and fighting, are flowing out. Continue in this manner for a number of breaths, visualizing, or mentally enumerating, the positives coming in and negatives going out.

Personal Wizard

Imagine an all powerful wizard. His robes are flowing; his beard is long and white. This wizard is very wise with powerful magic. He will give you advice to help solve problems. He can grant you special powers. He can take away troubling feelings. Allow the wizard to work his magic in your life.

Perspective

Imagine you are a bird taking flight. You sweep up into the sky, soaring high above. Look down. What can you see? Explore the houses, buildings, and streets. The people appear as tiny dots. Fly higher. Buildings and trees shrink. Eventually all you can see beneath you is the world as a small, revolving ball hovering in space. From here, visualize your problems as a speck of dust on the earth below you. Think how the wind will pick it up and blow it far away.

Rainbow Countdown

Make your mind blank, like a dark, very large TV screen. Now picture a red number 7 on your TV screen. Hold it there for a moment, and then let it float away, out of sight, as you replace it with an orange 6. Repeat in sequence with a yellow 5, a green 4, a blue 3, an indigo 2 and a purple 1. After the 1 has gone, let your mind return to the large blank TV screen.

Special Symbols

As you relax, allow your mind to drift. You are looking for something special: a unique object or symbol from deep within. This object will help you to remember things you need to remember, or let go of something distressing. It may allow you to be courageous, to find your voice, or to be relaxed and calm. Allow your imagination to fill in all the details of this symbol, its colour, shape, and size. Let this symbol rest in your heart and bring it to mind anytime you need to.

Tense and Release

Tighten the muscles in your feet. Really clench them, then let go. Feel your feet relax completely. Now tighten your feet, then your legs. Release and breathe. This time start with the feet, add the legs & buttocks. Squeeze, then let go. Once again, start with the feet, legs, buttocks and torso. Really contract those muscles. Then relax them completely. Now tighten the feet, legs, buttocks, torso, and arms. Squeeze those hands tight. Last time—start with your feet, next legs, buttocks, torso, arms, and face.

Tense your entire body, hold it tight, and release. Enjoy the feeling of complete relaxation from head to toe.

Walk in the Park

Bring to your mind's eye a beautiful city park. As you walk along a path through the trees, become aware of the texture of the ground beneath you. Enjoy the breeze on your face. Smell the freshly mowed grass, or the newly fallen leaves. Listen for the sounds: birds chirping, crickets singing, children playing, water trickling from a fountain. Look up through the canopy of leaves, enjoy the glow of the golden sunlight as it filters through, and breathe deeply.

Waves

Imagine you are lying on the beach. The warm sand feels so comfortable on your back. The sun is warming your entire body. As you inhale, listen! It sounds like the waves coming up on to the shore. As you exhale, imagine the waves retreating to the sea. Keep breathing with the waves. Allow the wave of breath to fill your belly, then your chest, and then leave your belly, followed by your chest. Relax and enjoy.

Chapter 7   Fun with Yoga

I like nonsense; it wakes up the brain cells. Fantasy is a necessary ingredient in living, it's a way of looking at life through the wrong end of a telescope ... and that enables you to laugh at life's realities. — Theodore Geisel

Creative Exercises

Enjoying life is something kids do best. A baby's laugh is one of life's most natural and heartfelt reactions. Children love to play, romp, and have fun. As adults, we become more self-conscious, cynical, project-oriented, and often lose the ability to let go and enjoy the moment with pure abandon. This section taps into the child within. It includes numerous activities that build upon yogic foundations while providing room for personal expression and creativity. So go ahead, have some fun, laugh a little, and enjoy all that life has to offer.

Bicycle

Ride an imaginary bicycle by lying on your back, pedalling with legs in the air. After a short flat ride, add in hills. While going up, make sure to slow down the pedalling with the effort required to climb. And when you come down, open your legs wide and shout "wheeeeeee!"

Body Talk

In pairs, ask children to talk to each other without using words. See how easily messages can be sent with only body language. Give a few examples such as "Come here," "Wait a minute," "I'm tired," "Good job!"

Elephant Walk

Stand in a line one behind the other. Bend over and reach your right arm back through your legs. Catch the left hand of the person behind you. You are now holding their trunk and they are holding your tail. Walk slowly like a herd of elephants around the room, trying to stay connected.

Mirror, Mirror

In pairs, ask the children to copy one another. Stand facing your partner. Whoever goes first does an action slowly; their partner mimics, trying to match them like a reflection. Continue on for a minute, then switch roles. Once students get good at doing this slowly, do it at normal speed, then quickly for those with really good reflexes.

Roller Coaster

Sit on the floor in a row, one passenger behind another with your legs stretched out beside the forward person. Take a roller coaster ride with the first person leading the ride. Include dips, climbs, and corners, leaning left and right.

Train (Individual)

Sit cross-legged and use your arms as the wheels of a steam engine, fists closed, bent at ninety degrees, pumping at your sides. As your arms pump, make train noises "choo, choo, choo, choo." Go slower and faster. Have students become aware of their breath, the movement of the diaphragm, belly, and lungs. End with a long, loud train whistle, "Whoo, hoo!" while pulling down on the cord.

> The creative is the place where no one else has ever been. You have to leave the city of your comfort and go into the wilderness of your intuition. What you'll discover will be wonderful. What you'll discover is yourself.
> — Alan Alda

Train (Group)

Stand in a line together holding onto the person in front of you near their waist to make a Human Train. Go around the room like this, trying to maintain the connection to the person in front of you. Vary the speed, drop or pick up passengers or cargo as you go, twist and turn, go over hills or bridges (any obstacle like a bench or mat), and be sure to make lots of train noises. Allowing different students to be the conductor, the engine, and the caboose each time is most effective.

Tricky Tree

This is a version of **Tree** pose performed with a partner. Partners face one other and, instead of putting their foot on their own leg when performing **Tree** pose, they give their raised foot to their partner to hold. The finished pose resembles a capital H. This is very tricky for pre-schoolers who are just learning to balance.

Games and Activities

Add One

This is a memory game where you build a sequence one pose at a time. The first person does a pose. The group does the first pose and the second person adds another one. The group repeats the first and second poses, and then the third person adds a new, different pose to the chain. Continue on (working as a group to remember the order) until all students have had a chance to add a pose.

Freeze Dance

Play some fun music and have everyone dance around the room. When the music stops, everyone must freeze in a yoga pose. The teacher may then go around and give suggestions on how to better perform the pose. Suggesting a few poses before starting always helps. Encourage the students to perform a different pose each time the music stops.

Hunters and Bears

Divide the children into two groups: bears and hunters. The children act out the movements as they listen to the story.

A **hunter** goes out to the woods on a bear hunt (walk in place).

He hears a **bear** roaring (roar).

The **hunter** drops his gun in fright (stamp feet on floor).

The **bear** comes closer and closer (crawl toward hunter).

The **hunter** drops to the ground and pretends to be dead (lie very still on floor)

The **bear** investigates the hunter to see whether he is alive (snuggle around the hunter).

The **hunter** must not laugh (be very quiet).

Fooled by the clever hunter, the **bear** walks away (crawl away).

Invent a Pose

This is often used when children want or need to express an idea or object but there is no official yoga pose for it. Tell them the pose doesn't exist until they create it. Encourage students to follow their first instinct and let their intuition lead them. For example, in the story **Farmyard Fun** (p.32), students often suggest 'sheep' or 'pig.' There are no such *asanas* but students are terrific at improvising to create one. You also can do this as its own activity, allowing students to invent 'spider pose,' 'waterfall pose,' 'happy pose,' 'strong pose,' etc.

Mother May I?

One child is the 'Mother' and stands at the front of the group. Children ask "Mother, may I be a ___(yoga pose)___?" The 'Mother' responds either, "Yes," and everyone performs the pose, or, "No, but you can be a (different yoga pose)," and everyone performs the pose 'Mother' suggests.

Name this Pose

Have students come into a familiar pose. Invite them to observe how they feel in the pose, and what thoughts and images come to mind as they hold the pose. Tell students to 'name' the pose, based on their experience. After, come into a resting pose. For example, while performing **Chair** pose, students may come up with "legs tired pose" or "flame reaching pose". After sharing their new pose name, students rest in **Child's** pose until all have finished.

> ## If you want creative workers, give them enough time to play.
> — John Cleese

Opposites

Have students come into a familiar pose. Then ask them to practise the 'opposite' pose. Don't tell them what the opposite pose is but instead invite them to make a pose that seems to have an opposite quality. You may find that students may flip a pose upside down, turn an active pose into a passive pose, or perform an actual yoga counter pose. Be prepared for interesting personal interpretation. Performing four to six poses in a row in this manner is a great exercise, and provides good discussion or journalling material.

Rowing in Unison

This is a wonderful listening game. Everyone sits on the floor. When the teacher says "toes," reach forward, and "back," lean back, with everyone following in unison. Switch it up to see if everyone is listening.

Choose a new caller from the group and repeat.

Swami Says

Similar to Simon Says. One person is the 'Swami' and stands at the front of the group. When the 'Swami' says, "Swami says, (yoga pose) ," everyone needs to do it. If the 'Swami' only says, " (yoga pose) ," anyone who does the pose is out.

Sea Shells

Divide playing area into two. Designate one area as the Sea, another as the Shore. Children run around both areas. When the teacher says "Sea," all the children run to that area. When the teacher says "Shore," they run to that area. When the teacher says "Shells," children stop and perform a yoga pose.

Teacher's Puppet

Let one child sit on your lap and pretend they are teaching. Gently hold their wrists and move their arms in an animated way while you describe the next pose. Use different voices and accents or try hand gestures like scratching their head or blowing kisses. This is very popular, and students will jump into your lap for a turn each time you sit down.

Yoga Tag

A form of Freeze Tag where, when 'It' tags you, you must perform a yoga pose. Any students not frozen can un-freeze you by running or crawling under part of the body. Each time you are frozen, you must perform a different yoga pose.

Letter to Parents

DATE: _____

Dear Parents,

This year our class will be doing yoga as part of our physical activities. We will be focusing on *Hatha* yoga, or physical yoga, which involves various physical poses, breathing exercises, and relaxation techniques.

We are excited to offer yoga to our students for the many benefits it offers. These include:

- Increased flexibility
- Enhanced strength and resiliency
- Improved balance
- Greater ability to concentrate
- Improved breathing and lung capacity
- Increased body-awareness and self-image
- Reduced stress

We will be working with many of the stories, activities, and games outlined in *Once Upon a Pose: A Guide to Yoga Adventure Stories for Children* by Donna Freeman. The lessons presented in this book focus on the physical aspects of yoga practice, and correspond to many of the themes and topics our class is studying. Feel free to come peruse of copy of this book if you have any concerns about the content of the lessons.

If you have any questions, please contact me at the school at _____.

Sincerely,

Recommended Reading

Betts, Dion E. *Yoga for Children with Autism Spectrum Disorder: A Step-by-Step Guide for Parents and Caregivers*. Jessica Kingsley, 2006.

Carrol, Cain and Kimata, Lori. *Partner Yoga: Making Contact for Physical, Emotional and Spiritual Growth*. Rodale/Reach, 2000.

Chryssicas, Mary Kaye. *Breathe: Yoga for Teens*. DK, 2007.

Chryssicas, Mary Kaye. *I Love Yoga*. DK, 2005.

Fraser, Tara. *Total Yoga: A Step-by-step guide to yoga at home for everybody*. Duncan Baird, 2001, 2007.

Iyengar, B.K.S. *Light on Yoga*. Schocken Books, 1977.

Kaminoff, Leslie. *Yoga Anatomy*. Human Kinetics, 2007.

Krishnaswami, Uma. *The Happiest Tree: a Yoga Story*. Lee and Low Books, 2005.

Lavallée, Loise. *Du yoga avec Om'a*. Les editions du soleil de minuit, 2007.

Purperhart, Helen. *Yoga Zoo Adventure: Animal Poses and Games for Little Kids*. Hunter House, 2006.

Solis, Sydney. *Storytime Yoga:Teaching Yoga to Children through Story*. The Mythic Yogic Studio, 2007.

Solis, Sydney. *The Treasure in Your Heart: Yoga and Stories for Peaceful Children*. The Mythic Yoga Studio, 2007.

Sumar, Sonia. *Yoga for the Special Child: A Therapeutic Approach for Infants and Children with Down Syndrome, Cerebral Palsy and Learning Disabilities*. Special Yoga Publications, 1998.

Swami Vishnu-devnanada. *The Complete Illustrated Book of Yoga*. Bell New York, 1960.

Wenig, Marsha. *YogaKids: Educating the Whole Child Through Yoga*. Stewart, Tabori and Chang, 2003.

Resources

Organization	Website
Actions School BC	www.actionschoolsbc.ca
Alberta Education DPA	http://education.alberta.ca/teachers/resources/dpa.aspx
Ananda Yoga	www.ananadayoga.org
Anusara Yoga	www.anusara.com
Autism Society of Canada	www.autismsocietycanada.ca
Bikram Yoga	www.bikramyoga.com
British Columbia DPA	www.bced.gov.bc.ca/dpa/
Canadian Attention Deficit Hyperactivity Disorder Resource Alliance	www.caddra.ca
Canadian Lung Association	www.lung.ca
Cerebral Palsy Association of Alberta	www.cpalberta.com
Centre for ADD/ADHD Advocacy, Canada	www.caddac.ca
Down Syndrome Society	www.cdss.ca
Dr. Dean Ornish Program to Reversing Heart Disease	www.hsc.wvu.edu/wellness/ornish/
Ever Active Schools	www.everactive.org
Integral Yoga	www.iyiny.org
Iyengar Yoga	www.bksiyengar.com
Kripalu Yoga	www.kirpalu.org
Kundalini Yoga	www.kirya.org
Ontario DPA	www.edu.gov.on.ca/eng/teachers/dpa.html
Sivananda Yoga	www.sivananda.org
Storytime Yoga	www.storytimeyoga.com
Svaroopa Yoga	www.svaroopayoga.org
Viniyoga	www.viniyoga.com
World Wildlife Federation	www.worldwildlife.org
Yoga for the Special Child	www.specialyoga.com
Yoga in My School	www.yogainmyschool.com
Yoga Journal	www.yogajournal.com
YogaKids	www.yogakids.com

Glossary

Affirmation	declaration that something is true; a positive assertion which develops positive outcomes
Ahimsa	non-violence: an attitude of not wanting to harm any living being, including yourself, in work, thought, or action
Ananda yoga	gentle, classic style of yoga founded by Swami Kriyananda; an inwardly directed practice which includes energizing exercises and affirmations; based upon the teachings of Paramhansa Yogananda, author of *Autobiography of a Yogi*
Anusara yoga	school of *Hatha* yoga founded by John Friend in 1997, which unifies a life-affirming Tantric philosophy of intrinsic goodness with Universal Principles of Alignment
Aparigraha	avoiding greed: non-possessiveness, limiting your possessions to what is necessary or important
Asana	physical postures or poses; one of the Eight Limbs of Yoga; ideally a comfortable and steady posture; discipline of the body
Ashtanga yoga	vigorous style of yoga aimed at building strength and stamina; also known as Power Yoga
Asteya	not stealing: take and use only that which is freely given, do not indulge in jealousy or covet others' possessions
Aum	a mythical or sacred symbol; used at the beginning and end of most mantras
Bhakti yoga	the path of highest spiritual attainment through systemized devotion, poetry, dance, and music; a religious experience offered to anyone, anywhere at anytime
Bikram Choudhury	founder of Bikram yoga
Bikram yoga	copyrighted series of 26 asanas that are performed in a hot environment; also known as Hot yoga
B.K.S. Iyengar	founder of Iyengar yoga; considered one of the foremost yoga teachers in the world and has been practicing and teaching yoga for more than 75 years; author of *Light on Yoga, Light on Pranayama*, and *Light on the Yoga Sutras of Patañjali*
Brahmacarya	conservation: living a life of moral restraint, controlling your senses, avoiding over-indulgences, understanding that true joy cannot be found in material or sensual pleasures
Dean Ornish	founder and president of the non-profit Preventive Medicine Research Institute in Sausalito, CA; author of six best-selling books; directed clinical research demonstrating, for the first time, that comprehensive lifestyle changes may begin to reverse even severe coronary heart disease, without drugs or surgery

Dharana	concentration upon a physical object, one of the Eight Limbs of yoga
Dhyana	meditation, undisturbed flow of thought, one of the Eight Limbs of yoga
Drishti	view or sight; a focal point used with *asanas* or meditation; helps focus the mind and develops concentration by eliminating visual distractions; encourages inner and outer balance
Hatha	derived from the words *ha* and *tha* meaning sun and moon, a strong practice used to purify; what most people in the West associate with yoga
Howard Gardner	psychologist at Harvard University best known for his theory of multiple intelligences
Integral yoga	developed by Swami Satchidanada as an integration of *karma, jnana,* and *bhakti* yoga in order to develop every aspect of the individual: physical, intellectual, and spiritual
Ishvara pranidhana	surrender: letting go of preconceived notions of self, others, and situations
Iyengar yoga	style of yoga developed by B.K.S. Iyengar and focusing on precise alignment of the body during *asanas*
Jnana yoga	the path of knowledge; knowing the body and the soul; gaining salvation through six virtues: control of the mind, control of the senses, renunciation of activities that are not duties, endurance, faith, and perfect concentration
John Friend	founder of Anusara yoga; produced numerous books, DVDs and CDs; a charismatic and respected *Hatha* yoga teacher
K. Pattabhi Jois	an Indian yoga teacher and student of Sri T. Krishnamacharya; established the Ashtanga Yoga Research Institute, which attracts thousands of foreign yoga students every year
Karma yoga	discipline of action; selfless love and service without thought for reward or recognition
Kripalu yoga	a therapeutic and spiritually focused practice which emphasizes compassionate self-acceptance, observing the activity of the mind without judgment, and taking what is learned into daily life; trademark of the Kripalu Yoga Fellowship
Kundalini	corporeal energy or an unconscious, instinctive force envisioned either as a goddess or a sleeping serpent coiled at the base of the spine; considered a part of the subtle body along with *chakras* (energy centres) and *nadis* (channels)
Kundalini yoga	a physical and meditative discipline; sometimes called 'yoga of awareness' because it awakens the *kundalini*, which is the unlimited potential that already exists within every human being
Mantra yoga	origins in Vedic Sciences and Tantra; it is said that any person who can chant or sing Vedas can achieve the ultimate salvation or union with supreme consciousness by chanting the mantras

Mary Kaye Chryssicas	yoga instructor and author of *I Love Yoga, Breathe: Yoga for Teens,* and the *Yoga for Teens Card Deck*
Marsha Wenig	yoga instructor and founder of YogaKids
Namaste	a common spoken greeting or salutation meaning "I bow to you"
Niyama	observances; one of the Eight Limbs of yoga by Patañjali
Patañjali	author of the yoga sutras dating from the 2nd century BC
Prana	Sanskrit word for breath; a life-sustaining force of living beings and vital energy
Pranayama	breath control; one of the Eight Limbs of yoga; beneficial to health, steadies the body and is highly conducive to the concentration of the mind
Pratyahara	sense withdrawal; one of the Eight Limbs of yoga
Rama Berch	creator of Svaroopa yoga; founder of Master Yoga Foundation, and founding president of Yoga Alliance, the US national non-profit organization that sets standards for and fosters integrity within the yoga community
Raja yoga	royal yoga; also known as Classical yoga; one of the six orthodox schools of Hindu philosophy; outlined by the sage Patañjali in his *Yoga Sutras*; concerned principally with the cultivation of the mind using meditation to further one's acquaintance with reality to finally achieve liberation
Samadhi	self-realization; one of the Eight Limbs of yoga; oneness with the object of meditation
Sanskrit	historical Indo-Aryan language and one of the 22 official languages of India
Santosha	contentment: being happy with who you are, where you are, and with what you have
Saucha	cleanliness: taking care to have a clean body and environment; developing a life based on a foundation of pure actions, words, and thoughts
Satya	honesty: ultimate truth; being true to and honest with yourself and those you encounter
Sivananda	Hindu spiritual teacher and a well-known proponent of yoga; founder of The Divine Life Society and author of over 200 books on yoga, vedanta and a variety of other subjects; established Sivananda Ashram on the bank of the Ganges
Sri T Krishnamacharya	influential Indian yoga teacher, healer, and scholar; students include many of today's most influential teachers: B.K.S. Iyengar, K. Pattabhi Jois, Indra Devi, Srivatsa Ramaswami, and Krishnamacharya's own sons T.K. Srinivasan, T.K.V. Desikachar and T.K. Sribhashyam; developed a vigorous style of yoga aimed at building strength and stamina that is known today as the popular Ashtanga (Vinyasa) Yoga
Sthira	Sanskrit word meaning solid, durable, strong, compact

Sukha	Sanskrit word meaning easy, pleasant, gentle, agreeable
Svaroopa yoga	style of yoga developed by Rama Berch and based on spinal openings; name is derived from a Sanskrit word meaning you know yourself at the deepest level of your being
Swami Kriyananda	founder of Ananda yoga; disciple of Paramhansa Yogananda; spiritual leader and founder of the Ananda Communities; author of numerous books
Swami Satchidananda	Indian religious figure, spiritual teacher and yoga adept, who became influential in the US; the founder of the Integral Yoga Institute and, in 1986, opened the Light of Truth Universal Shrine (LOTUS) at Yogaville in Virginia
Sonia Sumar	founder of Yoga for the Special Child, yoga instructor, author of *Yoga for the Special Children: A Therapeutic Approach to Infants and Children with Down Syndrome, Cerebral Palsy, and Learning Disabilities*
Svadhyaya	worthwhile study and learning: lifelong learning and being open to new ideas and approaches
Sydney Solis	storyteller and yoga instructor, author of *Storytime Yoga*, and *The Treasure in Your Heart: Yoga and Stories for Peaceful Children*
Tapas	self-discipline: keeping the body fit and well-functioning; making the most of yourself; setting goals and not giving up easily
T.K.V. Desikachar	son and student of Sri T. Krishnamacharya; established Krishnamacharya Yoga Mandiram, a leading centre of yoga and yoga studies in Chennai, India; books include *Health, Healing and Beyond, The Heart of Yoga: Developing a Personal Practice,* and *Viniyoga of Yoga*
Viniyoga	used by T.K.V. Desikachar to describe his approach and conviction that yoga practice should be adapted to fit the individuality and particular situation of each individual
Vishu-devananda	disciple of Swami Sivananda and founder of the International Sivananda Yoga Vedanta Centres and Ashrams; brought yoga to the west in the 1960s; considered an authority on *Hatha* and *Raja* yoga; the author of *The Complete Illustrated Book of Yoga*
Yama	restraints; one of the Eight Limbs of yoga by Patañjali
Yoga	traditional mental and physical disciplines originating in India; outside India, the term typically refers to *Hatha* yoga and its *asanas*
YogaKids	method of teaching yoga to children developed by Marsha Wenig
Yoga Sutras	an enormously influential work on yoga philosophy and practice dating from the 2nd century BCE; defines the best yoga practices, presenting these as the Eight Limbs

Indexes
Asanas – Translations

English	French	Sanskrit	Page
Back-to-Back Rises	Élévations arrière dos-à-dos		70
Basic Training	Formation de base		70
Bear Walk	Marcher comme un ours		71
Boat	Le bateau	Navasana	71
Bumble Bee Lips	Lèvres d'abeille		72
Bus	L'autobus		72
Camel	Le chameau	Ustrasana	73
Cat	Le chat	Marjarasana	73
Chair	La chaise	Utkatasana	74
Child's	L'enfant	Balasana	74
Cobbler's	Le cordonnier	Baddha konasana	75
Cobra	Le cobra	Bhujangasana	75
Compass	La boussole		76
Corpse	Le cadavre	Savasana	77
Cow-Faced	Le visage de la vache	Gomukhasana	77
Crocodile	Le crocodile	Chataranga	78
Crow	Le corbeau	Bakasana	78
Dancer	Le roi de la danse	Natarajasana	79
Deer	Le cerf	Marichiyasana II	79
Dolphin	Le dauphin		80
Donkey Kicks	Coup de sabots de l'âne		80
Downward Dog	Le chien à la baisse	Adho mukha svanasana	81
Eagle	L'aigle	Garudasana	81
Elephant	L'éléphant		82
Fish	Le poisson	Matsyasana	82
Gate	Le portail	Parighasana	83
Growing Flower	La fleur croissante		83
Half Moon	La demi-lune	Ardha chandrasana	84
Happy Baby	Le bébé très heureux	Ananda Balasana	84
Hero	Le héros	Virasana	85
Inchworm	L'arpenteuse		85
King Cobra	Le cobra royal	Bhujangasana	86
Lion	Le lion	Simhasana	86

Locust	La locuste	Salabhasana	87
Lotus	Le lotus	Padmasana	87
Monkey	Le singe		88
Moon Buggy	Le véhicule lunaire		88
Moon Walk	Promenade sur la lune		89
Mountain	La montagne	Tadasana	89
Phone	Le téléphone		90
Pigeon	Le pigeon	Eka pada rajakapotasana	90
Plough	La charrue	Halasana	91
Pyramid	La pyramide	Parsvottanasana	91
Rabbit	Le lapin	Sasangasana	92
Ragdoll	La poupée de chiffon		92
Robot	Le robot		93
Rock the Baby	Bercer l'enfant		93
Rocket	La fusée		94
Shower	Prendre une douche		94
Sphinx	Le sphinx		95
Spider	L'araignée		95
Star (body)	L'étoile (le corps)		96
Star (hand)	L'étoile (la main)		96
Tent	La tente	Prasarita Padottanasana	97
Tiptoe	La pointe des pieds		97
Tree	L'arbre	Vriksasana	98
Turtle	La tortue	Kurmasana	98
Two Scoops	Deux boules de crème glacée		99
Warrior	Le guerrier	Virabhadrasana II	99
Washing Machine	La machine à laver		100
Wheel	La roue	Urdva dhanurasana	100

Asanas – Stories

English	Story
Back-to-Back Rises	Farmyard Fun (p.32)
Basic Training	Man on the Moon (p.36)
Bear Walk	Mountain Magic (p.38)
Boat	Sailing, Sailing (p.40), Trip Down the Nile (p.44)
Bumble Bee Lips	Crawling and Flying (p.28), Garden Delights (p.34)
Bus	Mountain Magic (p.38)
Camel	Tour of India (p.42), Trip Down the Nile (p.44)
Cat	Family Time (p.30), Farmyard Fun (p.32), Trip Down the Nile (p.44)
Chair	African Safari (p.26), Tour of India (p.42)
Child's	Family Time (p.30), Garden Delights (p.34)
Cobbler's	Garden Delights (p.34), Mountain Magic (p.38)
Cobra	African Safari(p.26), Tour of India (p.42)
Compass	Man on the Moon (p.36), Sailing, Sailing (p.40)
Corpse	All
Cow-Faced	Farmyard Fun (p.32), Tour of India (p.42)
Crocodile	Crawling and Flying (p.28), Tour of India (p.42), Trip Down the Nile (p.44)
Crow	Crawling and Flying (p.28), Farmyard Fun (p.32)
Dancer	African Safari (p.26)
Deer	African Safari (p.26), Mountain Magic (p.38)
Dolphin	Sailing, Sailing (p.40)
Donkey Kicks	Farmyard Fun (p.32)
Downward Dog	Family Time (p.30), Farmyard Fun (p.32)
Eagle	Crawling and Flying (p.28), Mountain Magic (p.38), Sailing, Sailing (p.40), Trip Down the Nile (p.44)
Elephant	African Safari (p.26)
Fish	Garden Delights (p.34), Sailing, Sailing (p.40)
Gate	Farmyard Fun (p.32)
Growing Flower	Crawling and Flying (p.28)
Half Moon	Garden Delights (p.34), Man on the Moon (p.36), Sailing, Sailing (p.40)
Happy Baby	African Safari (p.26), Family Time (p.30)
Hero	African Safari (p.26)
Inchworm	Crawling and Flying (p.28), Garden Delights (p.34)

Printed in the United States
By Bookmasters